ethics in practice:
moral theory and the professions

ANDREW ALEXANDRA holds a Bachelor of Philosophy from the University of Oxford and a Master of Arts in Philosophy from the University of Melbourne. He is Senior Research Fellow and Director of the Australian Research Council-funded Special Research Centre for Applied Philosophy and Public Ethics (CAPPE), University of Melbourne division. He has research interests and publications in the areas of professional and applied ethics, political philosophy, and the history of philosophy. He is the co-author of *Police Ethics* (2006) and *Reasons, Values and Institutions* (2002), and co-editor of *Private Military Companies: Ethics, Theory and Practice* (2008) and is editor of the *Australian Journal of Professional and Applied Ethics*. Alexandra has extensive teaching experience in undergraduate and postgraduate courses in ethical theory and professional ethics, including development of courses for police, nurses and social welfare workers.

SEUMAS MILLER is Professor of Philosophy at Charles Sturt University and the Australian National University (joint position). He was Foundation Director of CAPPE (2000–07) and is currently Director of the ANU division of the centre. He is also Senior Research Fellow in Philosophy at the Centre for Ethics and Technology at Delft University of Technology. Miller has authored or co-authored 10 books, including *Social Action: A Teleological Account* (2001), *Corruption and Anti-Corruption* (2005) and *Moral Foundations of Social Institutions* (2009). He is the author or co-author of over 100 refereed academic articles. Miller has undertaken numerous consultancies, including for the Professional Standards Council, the Independent Commission Against Corruption, AusAID, the Department of the Prime Minister and Cabinet, the Australian Taxation Office, IBM (Europe) and the government of India.

To Mary

ethics in practice: moral theory and the professions

Andrew
Alexandra
and
Seumas
Miller

UNSW PRESS

A UNSW Press book

Published by
University of New South Wales Press Ltd
University of New South Wales
Sydney NSW 2052
AUSTRALIA
www.unswpress.com.au

© Andrew Alexandra and Seumas Miller 2009
First published 2009

National Library of Australia
Cataloguing-in-Publication entry
        Author: Alexandra, Andrew
        Title: Ethics in practice: moral theory and the professions
        Andrew Alexandra and Seumas Miller.
        ISBN: 978 1 74223 030 6 (pbk.)
        Notes: Includes index.
            Bibliography.
        Subjects: Ethics.
           Professional ethics.
           Work ethic.
        Other Authors/Contributors: Miller, Seumas
        Dewey Number: 174

Design Di Quick
Cover iStock
Printer Ligare

This book is printed on paper using fibre supplied from plantation or
sustainably managed forests.

Contents

Preface

This is a work of applied philosophy, reflecting our experience of the ways philosophical theory and empirical research can illuminate each other. It draws together and refines scholarly and original applied research work undertaken by the authors, individually and jointly, on a range of topics in professional and practical ethics. These include the relationship between moral theory and practice, the nature of professions and professional role morality, collective responsibility, and specific moral controversies over issues such as filial duty, euthanasia and recreational drug use. Our research on these matters – and our approach to presenting this research to students and practitioners – has been developed and tested through our involvement in three different, though related, kinds of activities. The first is our teaching of ethics to students in professional courses, including policing, nursing, and social welfare, as well to philosophy students in applied ethics subjects. The second is our collaboration with professional groups in research projects and consultancies. These groups include social workers, police officers, health and safety professionals, and professional associations. The third is our presentation and discussion of our ideas in academic settings such as seminars, and their publication in journals and books.

In each of these settings we have accrued intellectual and personal debts, too numerous to acknowledge in more than general terms here. We have had the good fortune over the past decade to work in the Australian Research Council Special Research Centre for Applied Philosophy and Public Ethics, a setting which has allowed us to interact with first-rate philosophers. We are grateful for the helpfulness, efficiency and forbearance of the staff at UNSW Press, and in particular for the guidance of our editor, Jessica Perini. Thanks are also due to Ewen Miller and Ned Dobos for their help in preparing the manuscript for publication, and to Wendy Bowles and John Blackler for providing some of the case studies we used.

Earlier versions of some of the material in this book appeared in the following previously published works. Andrew Alexandra: (2000) 'Dirty Harry and dirty hands' in Tony Coady, Steve James, Seumas Miller and Michael O'Keefe (eds) *Violence and Police Culture*, Melbourne University Press, Melbourne, pp 235–48. Andrew Alexandra, Steve Matthews and Seumas Miller: (2002) *Reasons, Values and Institutions*, Tertiary Press, Croydon. Andrew Alexandra and Seumas Miller: (2003) 'Needs, moral self-consciousness and professional roles' in John Rowan and Samuel Zinaich (eds) *Ethics for the Professions*, Wadsworth, Belmont, pp 134–40; (2005) 'Common morality and "institution-alising" ethics', *Australian Journal of Professional and Applied Ethics*, vol 7, no 1, pp 24–33; (2009) 'Ethical theory, "common morality" and professional obligations', *Theoretical Medicine and Bioethics*, vol 30, no 1, pp 69–80. Andrew Alexandra and Ann Woodruff: (2002) 'A code of ethics for Australian nurses' in Sidney Bloch and Margaret Coady (eds) *Codes of Ethics in the Professions*, Melbourne University Press, Melbourne, pp 226–43. Michael Collingridge and Seumas Miller: (1997) 'Filial responsibility and the care of the aged', *Journal of Applied Philosophy*, vol 14, no 2, p 123. Michael Collingridge, Seumas Miller and Wendy Bowles: (2001) 'Privacy and confidentiality in social work', *Australian Social Work*, vol 54(2), pp 3–14. Seumas Miller: (2001) *Social Action: A Teleological Account*, Cambridge University Press, New York; (2005) 'Individual autonomy and sociality' in Fred Schmitt (ed) *Socializing Metaphysics*, Rowman Littlefield, Oxford, pp 271–74; (2006) 'Collective moral responsibility' in Peter French and Howard Wettstein (eds) *Midwest Studies in Philosophy*, vol XXX; (2008) *Terrorism and*

Counter-terrorism, Blackwell, Oxford; (2005) 'Corruption', *Stanford Encyclopaedia of Philosophy*; (2009) *Moral Foundations of Social Institutions*, Cambridge University Press, New York. Seumas Miller, John Blackler and Andrew Alexandra: (2006) *Police Ethics*, 2nd edition, Allen & Unwin, Sydney. Seumas Miller, Edward Spence and Peter Roberts: (2005) *Corruption and Anti-Corruption*, Prentice Hall, Upper Saddle River.

This list should not be taken to imply that this work is only accessible to those with a background in philosophy. Philosophical jargon and technicalities have been kept to a minimum. We hope that anyone who is prepared to think seriously about the topics we discuss will be assisted in doing so by this book.

1: Ethical theory and practice

On Boxing Day 2004, a tsunami smashed into coastal communities around the Indian Ocean, killing hundreds of thousands and leaving many more in desperate need. Around the world, people responded with shock and sympathy, immediately moving to assist victims of the disaster. Charities raised huge amounts; volunteers risked their own lives and wellbeing to work in disease-ridden and dangerous locations.

Events such as these demonstrate a number of important aspects of morality. (A terminological point: throughout this book we use 'ethics' and 'morality' interchangeably.) Firstly, they show how deeply rooted the moral impulse is. People were profoundly moved, and motivated by the plight of others whom they had never met and who were remote from them geographically and culturally. Secondly, they show that many moral judgments are uncontroversial and easy to make. It was natural for people to feel for the victims of the tsunami. Conversely, anyone who understood the havoc the tsunami caused and did not care about it would be callous. Donors acted well; the volunteers who risked their own wellbeing to assist others were heroic.

That the truth of claims like these is so obvious – indeed so apparent as to generally go without saying – indicates the way moral-ity is largely 'second nature' for us. Dozens of times a day, in matters both grave and mundane, our actions and judgments are unhesitat-ingly guided by our sense of what is right or wrong, fair or unfair, kind or mean, and so on. And, mostly, no serious disagreement exists between people about the responses we make.

Still, against this background of the certainty and unanimity of many moral judgments, we find ourselves facing situations of moral complexity and uncertainty. Perhaps these are novel situations, cre-ated by the advance of technology. It seems good to help the infertile have children, but does that make reproductive cloning acceptable? Perhaps they are situations where values collide: it is good to be honest and good to be kind, but what should you do when answer-ing a question honestly will be hurtful? Sometimes it is even unclear whether something is a moral matter at all. Some people think that whether someone engages in sexual activity with members of their own sex rather than the opposite sex is merely a matter of personal taste, no more a moral issue than the choice of a cat rather than a dog for a pet; others claim that it is of great moral importance.

This book is written with a practical aim in mind: to assist the reader to make better informed, more rationally justifiable decisions about how to act, and judge the actions of others, where there are mor-ally hard choices to be made in their professional working life. Here we invoke the admittedly vague and contested distinction between the so-called professions and other occupations. The traditional profes-sions include doctors, lawyers, engineers, and accountants. The new or emerging professions would include journalists, social workers and nurses.

We focus on professional practice for two connected reasons. Firstly, the tasks that professionals (in our narrow sense) undertake are *essentially* moral. In the case of lawyers their defining occupa-tional role is the administration of justice, in the case of doctors, human health. In the human services, more generally, the aim of professional groups is to help people, to make their situation better. But, secondly, moral uncertainty often and predictably arises in the course of professional life, and unless the professional has some way of assessing the options that are open to them, they cannot know if they are fulfilling the requirements of their job. Obviously, a social worker should try to help his client have a better life. But what if it is only possible to get a client to stop engaging in activity that threatens their health by confining them against their will? Would the social worker be justified in being complicit in the infringement of their client's autonomy in such a situation? Furthermore, the demands of professional roles sometimes conflict with the demands of so-called 'ordinary morality', the morality that we generally apply in our dealings with each other. According to the demands of her role, a criminal lawyer is supposed to defend the interests of her client zealously. According to ordinary morality, we should not stand in the way of bringing serious criminals to justice. Should the lawyer then defend someone whom she believes is guilty of a serious crime and deserving of punishment?

The appropriate response to such questions is often not obvious. Rather, we have to reason about them: to try to understand what feasible courses of action are available to us, and to see the relevant reasons for and against these courses of action, and how much weight these reasons should be given. The fact that we often do not have to engage in difficult deliberation when we act morally does not mean that we act without reasons. In some cases, the reasons are so obvious that deliberation is unnecessary. On the other hand, in many cases, our understanding of the reasons may be implicit. We can feel their force, even if we do not spell out explicitly and in detail what they are and how we came to the conclusion we did. (Similarly, we may be perfectly competent at deciding which route to follow to get back home, who is a good footballer and who is not, whether we should buy a given house at the price being asked, and so on without providing ourselves or others with a worked out account of how we do so.)

Moral theory and moral theories

Making explicit the system underlying morality involves the construction of what might be called a moral theory. A theory gives a systematic, unified explanation for a range of phenomena. Thus, the theory of gravity posits the existence of a force that holds throughout the universe and applies to all physical objects. This is a powerful theory, since it helps us explain, and predict, a wide range of phenomena such as the trajectories of the planets in the solar system, the fact that rivers run to the sea, the movement of the tides, the falling of dropped balls, and so on; phenomena that, on the face of it, are very different in kind.

There does appear to be a system that underlies our moral thinking. It seems, for example, that we judge particular actions in the light of certain general moral principles. We may explain our anger at our friend by pointing out that they had broken a promise to meet us. Such an explanation presupposes that there is an accepted principle that we should keep promises. A moral theory, then, attempts to provide a way of identifying moral phenomena and to give a systematic, unified explanation of such phenomena.

Since morality is concerned with what we should do, a moral theory will be concerned with our actions. But the same action can be assessed in different ways.

Firstly, we may consider the *consequences* of the act; the desirable or undesirable things that follow from it. Consequences are important in our ordinary thinking about morality. We judge the drunk driver who kills a pedestrian much more harshly than the one who reaches home safely, and the only difference in their behaviour seems to be in the badness of its consequences. But consequences are not the only things we may take into account in judging an act; we may also look at the kind of act. Some acts are held to be good or bad in themselves, independently of their consequences. Lying is held to be bad, telling the truth good.

While the two most influential philosophical approaches to moral theory over the past few decades have both taken actions as the fundamental element in moral theory, they have differed from each other in which aspects of an action they consider to be basic. As the name implies, *consequentialist* moral theories hold that consequences are fundamental: ultimately, our actions are to be judged according to whether they may lead to the most desirable outcomes.

The most famous version of consequentialism is the classical utilitarianism propounded in the 19th century by the English philosopher, John Stuart Mill. In his work *Utilitarianism* (1863), Mill sharply distinguished between the moral rightness or wrongness of actions and the moral goodness or badness of persons. Mill regarded the Principle of Utility (originally formulated by Jeremy Bentham) as the guide to right action. According to this principle one should act so as to bring about 'the greatest happiness for the greatest number' (Bentham 1988). So an action is right if it tends towards the greatest happiness of the greatest number, and wrong if it does not. On Mill's account, ultimately all actions should be judged in the light of this principle.

Followers of such a doctrine could still hold that principles such as 'tell the truth', 'be kind' and so on, had moral force. But their force derives from the fact that generally following them was likely to contribute to bringing about the greatest happiness. Such principles, then, are more like rules of thumb: generally helpful guides to action, which should nevertheless be ignored when following them would conflict with producing the greatest happiness. 'Lying is wrong' is fine as a principle, just so long as following it *does* actually maximise the happiness of the greatest number of people. Where there is a conflict between the application of that principle and the Principle of Utility – where refusing to tell a lie would stand in the way of maximising happiness – then the principle of not lying loses its force. So an act of lying might be bad in one situation, because it has worse consequences than alternative available actions, and good in another, because lying in that situation produces the best consequences.

Other consequentialist moral theories differ from classical utilitarianism in seeing something other than happiness as the highest good. Some religious thinkers, for example, believe that we should aim to promote the word of God as much as possible. An action will be good, then, if it does this more effectively than any available alternative, and bad if it does not. (Henry Sidgwick (1907) provides a sophisticated and influential defence of utilitarianism; John Jamieson Carswe Smart and Bernard Williams (1973) argue (respectively) for and against it.)

Alternatively, deontological moral theories hold that the rightness or wrongness of an action rests, not on its consequences, but rather on the kind of action that it is. (The word 'deontology' derives from the Greek 'deon' for 'duty' and 'logos' meaning 'science of'.) Lying is, in itself, wrong, and telling the truth is, in itself, right. Hence we can know that an action is right (or wrong) without knowing anything about its consequences.

The great 18th century philosopher Immanuel Kant developed a particularly influential deontological theory. Kant thought that we could judge whether an action was morally permissible by appeal to the so-called Principle of Universalisability (Kant 1998). There are different renderings of this general principle, but in essence the idea is that one should only act on a specific maxim – or action guiding principle – if that maxim is one that could be consistently followed by everyone. Assume John is contemplating whether or not to lie to Bill about his (John's) financial situation, so that Bill will lend him some money. The relevant maxim is telling lies. Thus John must ask himself whether or not everyone could consistently adopt such a maxim. The answer to that is surely not. Lying can only be effective against a general presumption of trust. That presumption will hold only where most people aim to tell the truth most of the time, including when they could benefit from lying, or some other apparently good reason to do so exists. If everyone were disposed to lie whenever they thought there was a good reason to do so, the presumption of trust would soon be undermined, and with it both the possibility of benefiting from lying and indeed of meaningful communication itself. Therefore John does not want himself and everyone else to follow the maxim of telling lies. So he cannot consistently follow the maxim to tell lies. Therefore he ought not tell a lie on this occasion. It is morally wrong for him to tell this particular lie to Bill in virtue of the formal Principle of Universalisability.

One of the attractions of both the consequentialist and deontologist approaches is that they hold out the promise that whenever we are faced with a question about how to act there is, at least in principle, a method for generating the correct answer. On the other hand, both approaches to morality appear implausible by the lights of our ordinary way of thinking about morality. For the consequentialist, consequences (obviously) are all-important. He has no room for the thought that even if we believe that we did the right thing by, for example, lying, we may still regret having to tell a lie, and wish that we had not found ourselves in a situation where we felt that we should do so. While the utilitarian seems to give consequences too much weight, the deontologist arguably gives them too little. For her the fact that, for example, we could save a life by telling a lie is of no moral concern.

In our view it is illusory to seek an ethical theory that will deliver a single, unambiguous directive about how we should act in every difficult case. This is not to say that moral decision-making is not a matter of objective judgment, as opposed to subjective choice; far from it. However, moral truths are not delivered by mechanically applying a formula. Instead we need to take into account a range of relevant factors, including the nature of the action itself, but also such things as the likely consequences of the action, the motivation of the person involved, and so on. For example, though lying is, in itself, a bad thing, in some unusual cases it might be the right thing to do; for example when we can help avert a murder or some other great tragedy. In some cases there may not be a single obvious answer; perhaps whatever we do will be bad in some way; perhaps rational, morally good people may disagree about the best thing to do.

A central task of moral theory, as we see it, is to reveal the structure which underpins our moral judgments and practice, thereby helping us to become more self-conscious and critical in relation to the moral world in which we are already immersed. (For an explication and defence of this approach to moral theory see Gert 2004.) Our interest is in the way theoretical reflection on ethics can help us inform our thinking about particular practical problems. There can be no doubt of the relevance of moral theory to that task. For a start, as we indicate in the following chapters, many people are, more or less unconsciously, in the grip of some (perhaps imperfectly grasped) moral theory or other, and their responses to particular issues will perforce be influenced by those theories. If that theory is itself deficient, then many of their judgments are also likely to be faulty. More positively, a grasp of moral theory is likely to help us identify the major elements in morally complex situations, and reason more clearly about their relationship to each other. At the same time, our theoretical understanding must be tested through application to the reality of moral phenomena.

This understanding of the intertwined relationship of moral theory and practice has shaped the structure of this book. All our discussions arise from a focus on real, or at least realistic, 'case studies', drawn from history, literature, accounts of professional practice, and the like. These case studies are not contrived merely to illustrate some theoretical position. Rather, in the light of these case studies we test the usefulness and limits of the various theoretical positions and claims, while in the second half we deploy the insights gained to illuminate some of the distinctive practical ethical issues and problems commonly encountered by those who work in human services professions. The theoretical issues we consider include the question of whether morality is something that is determined by each society, the nature of moral principles, and of virtues and vices, and the characteristics of role morality. Informed consent, duty of care, euthanasia, the obligations of adult children to their parents, sexual morality, recreational drug taking, and corruption are among the practical issues we consider.

Readings

Aristotle (1973) *Nicomachean Ethics*, Thomson, James Alexander Kerr (translator), Penguin, Harmondsworth.

Bentham, Jeremy (1776, 1988) *A Fragment on Government*, Cambridge University Press, Cambridge.

Gert, Bernard (2004) *Common Morality: Deciding What to Do*, Oxford University Press, Oxford.

Kant, Immanuel (1785, 1998) *Groundwork of the Metaphysics of Morals*, Gregor, Mary (editor and translator), with an introduction by Korsgaard, Christine, Cambridge University Press, Cambridge.

—— (1788, 1997) *Critique of Practical Reason*, Gregor, Mary (editor and translator), with an introduction by Reath, Andrews, Cambridge University Press, Cambridge.

—— (1797, 1991) *The Metaphysics of Morals*, Gregor, Mary (translator), Cambridge University Press, Cambridge.

Mill, John Stuart (1863, 1998) *Utilitarianism*, Oxford University Press, Oxford (any edition).

Ross, William David (1930, 2002) *The Right and the Good*, Stratton-Lake, Philip (editor), Oxford University Press, New York.

Sidgwick, Henry (1907) *The Methods of Ethics*, 7th edition, Macmillan, London.

Smart, John Jamieson Carswe and Williams, Bernard (1973) *Utilitarianism: For and Against*, Cambridge University Press, Cambridge.

The Stanford Encyclopedia of Philosophy, available at <http://plato.stanford.edu> and *The Internet Encyclopedia of Philosophy*, available at <http://www.iep.utm.edu> (accessed 21/1/09).

2: Relativism

Everyone without exception believes his own native customs, and the religion he was brought up in, to be the best; and that being so, it is unlikely that anyone but a madman would mock at such things. There is abundant evidence that this is the universal feeling about the ancient customs of one's country. One might recall, in particular, an anecdote of Darius. When he was king of Persia, he summoned the Greeks who happened to be present at his court, and asked them what they would take to eat the dead bodies of their fathers. They replied that they would not do it for any money in the world. Later, in the presence of the Greeks, and through an interpreter, so they could understand what was said, he asked some Indians, of the tribe called Callatiae, who do in fact eat their parents' dead bodies, what they would take to burn them. They uttered a cry of horror and forbade him to mention such a dreadful thing. One can see by this what custom can do, and Pindar, in my opinion, was right when he called it 'king of all'.

Herodotus of Halicarnassus (1988) *The Histories*

CASE STUDY 2.2

[The following extract describes an anthropologist's observations of the behaviour of the Kwakiutl tribe of Indians in Canada.]

Fast Runner and Throw Away [two chiefs] were now in open enmity. They chose, therefore, to give rival initiations into the secret societies, using their religious privileges rather than their secular. Throw Away secretly planned to give this Winter Ceremonial, and Fast Runner, hearing of it through his informers, determined to outdo him. Throw Away initiated a son and a daughter, but Fast Runner two sons and two daughters. Fast Runner now had outdistanced his rival, and when his four children were brought back from their seclusion and the excitement of the dance was at its height, he had a slave scalped and butchered by the Fool dancers and the Grizzly Bear Society and the flesh eaten by the Cannibals. The scalp he gave to Throw Away, who clearly could not match this mighty deed.

Fast Runner had still another triumph. His daughters were being initiated as war dancers, and they asked to be put upon the fire. A great wall of firewood was raised about the fire, and the daughters were tied to boards ready to be committed to the flames. Instead, two slaves dressed like true war dancers and similarly tied to boards were put into the fire. For four days the daughters of Fast Runner remained in hiding, and then, from the ashes of the slaves which had been preserved, they apparently returned to life. Throw Away had nothing to match this great demonstration of privilege, and he and his men went off to fight the Nootka. Only one man returned to tell of the defeat and death of the war party ...

Ruth Benedict (1968) *Patterns of Culture*

CASE STUDY 2.3

[In this case study the same anthropologist discusses the behaviour of the Dobuans. Dobu is an island off the southern shore of New Guinea.]

A recent study of an island of north west Melanesia by [Reo] Fortune describes a society built upon traits which we regard as beyond the border of paranoia. In this tribe the exogamic groups look upon each other as prime manipulators of black magic, so that one marries always into an enemy group which remains for life one's deadly and unappeasable foes. They look upon a good garden crop as a confession of theft, for everyone is engaged in making magic to induce into his garden the productiveness of his neighbour's; therefore no secrecy in the island is so rigidly insisted upon as the secrecy of a man's harvesting of his yams. Their polite phrase at the acceptance of a gift is, 'And if you now poison me, how shall I repay you this present?' Their preoccupation with poisoning is constant; no woman ever leaves her cooking pot for a moment unattended. Even the great affinal economic exchanges that are characteristic of this Melanesian culture area are quite altered in Dobu since they are incompatible with this fear and distrust that pervades the culture … They go further and people the whole world outside their own quarters with such malignant spirits that all-night feasts and ceremonials simply do not occur here. They have even religiously enforced customs that forbid the sharing of seed even in one family group. Anyone else's food is deadly poison to you, so that communality of stores is out of the question. For some months before harvest the whole society is on the verge of starvation, but if one falls to the temptation and eats up one's seed yams, one is an outcast and a beachcomber for life. There is no coming back. It involves, as a matter of course, divorce and the breaking of all social rites.

Now in this society where no-one may work with another and no-one may share with another, Fortune describes the individual who was regarded by all his fellows as crazy. He was not one of those who periodically ran amok and, beside himself and frothing at the mouth, fell with a knife upon anyone he could reach. Such behaviour they did not regard as putting anyone outside the pale. They did not even put the individuals who were known to be liable to these attacks under any kind of control. They merely fled when they saw the attack coming on and kept out of the way. 'He would be all right tomorrow'. But there was one man of sunny, kindly disposition who liked work and liked to be helpful. The compulsion was too strong for him to repress it in favour of the opposite tendencies of his culture. Men and women never spoke of him without laughing; he was silly and simple and definitely crazy. Nevertheless, to the ethnologist used to a culture that has, in Christianity, made his type the model of all virtue, he seemed a pleasant fellow ...

It is a point that has been made more often in relation to ethics than in relation to psychiatry. We do not any longer make the mistake of deriving the morality of our own locality and decade directly from the inevitable constitution of human nature. We do not elevate it to the dignity of a first principle. We recognise that morality differs in every society, and is a convenient term for socially approved habits. Mankind has always preferred to say, 'It is morally good', rather than 'It is habitual', and the fact of this preference is matter enough for a critical science of ethics. But historically the two phrases are synonymous.

The concept of the normal is properly a variant of the concept of the good. It is that which society has approved. A normal action is one which falls well within the limits of expected behaviour for a particular society. Its variability among different peoples is essentially a function of the variability of the behaviour patterns that different societies have created for themselves, and can never be wholly divorced from a consideration of culturally institutionalised types of behaviour ...

Ruth Benedict (1934) 'Culture and the abnormal', *Journal of General Psychology*

CASE STUDY 2.4

[The Ik are an African tribe who live in the mountains of northeastern Uganda.]

In this curious society which seems to have bypassed Karl Marx in economics, there is one common value, apart from language, to which all Ik hold tenaciously. It is *ngag*, 'food'. This is not a cynical quip — there is no room for cynicism with the Ik. It is clearly stated by the Ik themselves in their daily conversation, in their rationale for action and thought. It is the one standard by which they measure right and wrong, goodness and badness. The very word for 'good', *marang*, is defined in terms of food. 'Goodness', *marangik*, is defined simply as 'food', and still further clarified as '*individual* possession of food'. Then if you try the word as an adjective and attempt to discover what their concept is of a 'good man', *iakw anamarang*, hoping that the answer will be that a good man is a man who helps you fill your own stomach, you get the truly Icien answer: a good man is one who *has* a full stomach. There is goodness in being, but none in doing, at least not in doing to others.

So we should not be surprised when the mother throws her child out at three years old. She has breast-fed it, with some ill humour, and cared for it in some manner for three whole years, and now it is ready to make its own way. I imagine the child must be rather relieved to be thrown out, for in the process of being cared for he or she is carried about in a hide sling wherever the mother goes, and since the mother is not strong herself this is done grudgingly. Whenever the mother finds a spot in which to gather, or if she is at a water hole or in her fields, she loosens the sling and lets the baby to the ground none too slowly, and of course laughs if it is hurt. I have seen Bila and Matsui do this many a time. Then she goes about her business, leaving the child there, almost hoping that some predator will come along and carry it off. This happened once while I was there — once that I know of, anyway — and the mother was delighted. She was rid of the child and no longer had to carry it about and feed it, and still further this meant that a leopard was in the vicinity and would be sleeping the child off and thus be an easy kill. The men set off and found the leopard, which had consumed all of the child except part of the skull; they killed the leopard and cooked it and ate it, child and all. That is Icien economy, and it makes sense in its own way. It does not, however, endear children to their parents or parents to their children.

Colin Turnbull (1972) *The Mountain People*

ETHICS IN PRACTICE

Aboriginal parents are, on the whole, very indulgent. They pet and spoil their children, and stand a great deal from them in the way of bad behaviour, or even disobedience. When they do punish it is likely to be severe – a sudden slap or a blow, when a mother or father loses patience: but punishment is rarely carried out in cold blood. In western Arnhem Land, drawing on a conventional theme from local mythology, a mother may threaten her child with a thrashing 'in spirit'. This means, simply, hitting his footprints or a tree, making a fine display of rage without touching him at all. It is a warning of what she *could do*, if provoked, but would prefer to avoid. The myths of this area contain many references to the danger of neglecting or ill-treating children: and in fact adults do go to some lengths to avoid denying them what they want. In north-eastern Arnhem Land a child who does not get his own way throws himself down on the ground in tantrums, writhing and kicking, crying or whimpering for hours at a time, ignored by everyone nearby, except that every now and then someone may turn and scream exasperation at him. A few girls continue to do this even after puberty. Boys have fewer opportunities for it after their first initiation rite, because from that point onward responsibility for disciplining them begins to pass from the boy's immediate family to the adult men of this particular *mada* and *mala*. But when a child is young, it is his own mother's or father's business to punish him – or not. Should someone else try, even a classificatory mother or father, or one of the father's other wives, or a grandparent, trouble is bound to ensue. If a mother rushes to help her little boy in a fight, and slaps his opponent, this can be the signal for a noisy encounter: other women come running to take sides, and the upshot may be a number of casualties. (Men, however, prefer to keep out of women's fights, unless their own interests are threatened).

Ronald and Catherine Berndt (1992) *The World of the First Australians: Aboriginal Traditional Life: Past and Present*

[In this case study, the Roman philosopher and statesman Marcus Tullius Cicero expresses his disapproval of the habits of the young men of Rome in the century before the birth of Christ.]

All of their interest in life and their waking hours are devoted to night-long banquets ... These boys, so delicate and soft, have learned not only to dance and sing, but also to wave daggers and sprinkle poisons. Unless they leave the city, unless they perish, be assured that in the state there will still be this hotbed of Catilines. But what do these wretches desire? They will not take with them to the camp their little mistresses, will they? Yet how can they be separated from them, especially on nights like these? How can these men endure the Apennines and that hoar-frost and snow? Unless they think perhaps that they will bear winter more easily because they have learned to dance naked at banquets!

Marcus Tullius Cicero (1937) *In Catilinam II*

ETHICAL ANALYSIS

The case studies present us with a number of odd, alien, even shocking forms of behaviour. Yet, apparently, within the cultures where they occur, they are seen as normal, unobjectionable, even morally desirable. We recoil in horror at the idea of having someone scalped, butchered and cannibalised; the Kwakiutl apparently see the willingness and ability to do this as a sign of someone's eminence. And as Herodotus reminds us in the story he tells in case study 2.1, members of the cultures at whose practices we look askance, are likely to take just the same attitude towards many of *our* practices. The Dobuans described in case study 2.3 would presumably find our idea of admirable character very strange.

These case studies graphically point to one of the most striking, and problematic, features of moral practice: what we'll call moral divergence. Moral divergence between cultures has excited thought and discussion since at least the time of Herodotus in the 5th century BC. In his day one of the major effects of the observation of moral divergence between cultures was to throw doubt on the idea that moral practices and responses were natural and necessary, in the way that the behaviour of physical objects is. Rather, moral behaviour came to be seen as something that was in some sense under human control, a matter of decision and choice.

Some thinkers, then and now, have drawn more radical conclusions from the fact of cultural divergence in moral matters. Some – moral nihilists – believe that the persistence of moral disagreement indicates that there are simply no moral truths to be known (Mackie 1977). If there were, surely there would have been general agreement by now. Others have been more cautious, hesitating to deny that there are moral truths. They think that the persistence of moral disagreement shows that, though some moral beliefs may well be true, we are not in a position to have any confidence as to which they are. These are the moral sceptics (Joyce 2001). Finally, there are those who have thought that moral claims may be true, but their truth (or falsity) is determined by their cultural context (Wong 1984; Benedict 1934). So the claim 'eating people is bad' is true for us, but false for cannibals. This view, that the truth or falsity of moral claims is relative to the beliefs current in a culture, is known, for obvious reasons, as 'cultural relativism'.

We will look at some of the theoretical issues surrounding cultural relativism in the following sections. For the moment, without denying the real differences between cultures, we wish to point out that these differences can be easily over-estimated. Consider, for example, Herodotus' story of the horrified reactions of the Greeks and Indians to being asked to treat the bodies of their fathers in a way which in the other culture is taken as a sign of piety. On the surface, it might look like the moral values of the two cultures are directly opposed. But in fact, the story shows that their values are significantly similar, since both agree that, rather than the bodies of dead fathers being simply discarded, they should be disposed of in a respectful manner. (Anthropologists have claimed that all cultures have some sort of funerary practice for the disposal of the dead.) Where they differ is in their views of the kinds of behaviour that manifest piety and impiety, not in the moral attitude which motivates their behaviour.

Similarly, behaviour which appears bizarre, unacceptable, even incomprehensible sometimes becomes much easier to understand, and the people engaged in it much less foreign to us, when we fill in the context of that behaviour. The attitude of the Ik towards their children, described in case study 2.4, strikes us on first reading as barely human. It becomes more understandable when their situation is explained. The Ik traditionally were a nomadic tribe, roaming over a large area of central Africa. In recent years, however, most of the lands over which they had ranged were turned into a national park, which they are forbidden to use. They were confined to a small and inhospitable area, facing drought conditions three out of every four years. Deprived of their traditional lands and way of life, in conditions of extreme hardship, most kinds of day-to-day cooperation disappeared from Ik society, as individuals fought for survival. Against this background what is surprising perhaps is not so much that mothers showed minimal concern for their children's wellbeing, but rather that they still showed *some* concern. Ik mothers, at the time described, still raised their children to the point where it was at least possible that they would be able to survive by fending for themselves – and in fact quite a number did survive – even though this was clearly at considerable personal cost. It would be difficult to be certain that mothers in our society are more self-sacrificing in the interests of their children than the Ik mothers.

Once we realise that the Ik live in dire necessity we find their behaviour much easier to understand. In fact we might behave in the same way if we found ourselves in a similar position. The behaviour of the Kwakiutl chiefs described in case study 2.2, on the other hand, surely will remain very alien to us no matter how extensively the background against which they act is filled in. It is surely impossible to seriously imagine that we could ever take pride in the butchering of a helpless human being, for example. But even here, the behaviour of the Kwakiutl is not totally alien to us. After all, we are familiar enough with competitive behaviour and conspicuous consumption, both of which the Kwakiutl display in a particularly brutal way. Furthermore, in cases like this we often find that the real difference between us and the members of other cultures lies not so much in our accepting radically different moral standards, but rather in our having different *factual* beliefs. The Kwakiutl may, for instance, believe that slaves are a lower form of life, so that taking their life is a much less serious matter than taking the life of free people. If they came to have the same factual beliefs as us – including the belief that slaves are persons with equal moral worth to that of free persons – their moral practices would appear much less different.

Case study 2.5, a sketch of the child-rearing practices of traditional Aborigines, illustrates the point that though the divergence in behaviour and attitudes is noteworthy, so is the considerable, and sometimes surprising, degree of cross-cultural similarity. Traditional Aborigines lived a nomadic life in small groups, without machines or writing, moving through a landscape they believed to be inhabited and shaped by spirit creatures. Their culture was about as different to that of modern European Australians as it is possible to imagine. Yet the attitudes to the raising and disciplining of children shown in the case study seem similar to those of our own. Similarly, in case study 2.6, we hear complaints familiar to us today about the supposed moral decay and self-indulgence of the 'youth of today' compared to their parents, but in this instance coming from the Roman statesman and philosopher Cicero over 2000 years ago.

Motivating cultural relativism

Above we looked at cases of moral difference between cultures. In the most extreme of these there seems to be a conflict in the judgments made in different cultures about the same sort of action. The Kwakiutl, it is claimed, regard the butchering of innocents in certain circumstances as admirable: we regard it as morally reprehensible. These views can be represented as claims about what is true. The Kwakiutl are claiming, in effect 'It is true that butchering people in circumstances C is morally good.' We are claiming in effect 'It is false that butchering people in circumstances C is good.' Since a claim cannot be true and false at the same time, at least one of these claims must be false. Which one?

Our attempt to answer this question is complicated by two considerations. The first is what we might call moral autonomy. Though there are people who we think of as more or less morally wise, virtually all mature human beings are capable of exercising independent moral judgment, and there must be a presumption that their judgment should be respected. This does not mean that we must agree with such judgments, but where we disagree with them, we should be prepared to argue the point, and if need be change our mind in the face of reasoned argument.

Furthermore – this is the second complicating factor – not only do moral beliefs often vary from culture to culture, the beliefs that people have are heavily influenced by their culture. If a Kwakiutl baby were brought up in modern Australia it would no doubt have the moral beliefs typical of modern Australians. Conversely if an Australian baby were brought up in Kwakiutl society, it would have the moral beliefs of that culture.

So there appears to be a symmetry in the position of members of, say, Kwakiutl and Australian cultures who hold opposing moral beliefs. The views of each demand to be taken with equal seriousness, and if each had been brought up in the other's culture they would probably hold the view with which they now disagree. Given the great disparity in world views between members of these cultures, it seems unlikely that either would be able to convince the other to their way of thinking. In most fields of human inquiry and practice we can turn to recognised experts for help in resolving disputed questions. In some cultures people can turn to moral authorities to provide moral advice. However, these authorities typically provide perspectives that are informed by the moral norms adhered to in that culture. But when it comes to moral disagreements between members of different cultures, who can resolve these arguments? There simply is no general agreement about one moral authority. Given this fact, there seems no way of resolving moral disagreements between members of such cultures by appealing to a third party.

The existence and persistence of moral disagreement poses a big problem for the idea that we can have moral knowledge. If, as argued in the last paragraph, opposed moral beliefs coming from different cultures have roughly equal claim to being true, what certainty can we have that what *we* take to be true, is? The cultural relativist believes that they have an answer to that question.

Defining cultural relativism

When a cannibal, say, claims 'Eating people is good' and an Australian asserts that 'Eating people is bad' we seem to have a direct contradiction. According to the cultural relativist there is no such contradiction. The cannibal should be understood as really saying 'The habit of eating people is approved of in our (cannibal) culture'; and the Australian as saying 'The habit of eating people is not approved of in our culture'. These two statements are about different subjects: one is about the case in cannibal culture, the other about the case in Australian culture. Since they have different subject matters they will not come into conflict, and in this case presumably they are both true.

The cultural relativist thinks that moral terminology is always at least implicitly relativised to particular cultures. The term 'morally good', for example, means 'approved of in the agent's (doer's) culture' and the term 'morally bad' means 'disapproved of in the agent's culture'. The truth or falsity of moral relativism depends on this claim about meaning. (There are in fact a number of slightly varying formulations of the cultural relativist understanding of the meaning of moral terms. Sometimes, as in Benedict's discussion in case study 2.2, it is put in terms of habitual behaviour. 'Good' would thus mean 'is habitually done in the speaker's society'. The strength of the position is not substantially affected by these differences.)

Cultural relativism needs to be subjected to philosophical scrutiny. Apart from anything else it is a widely, if somewhat inconsistently, held position. (Inconsistent because people often appeal to it when discussing other cultures, but don't apply it to moral issues in their own.) Furthermore it has a number of attractive features. As we have seen, it respects the moral claims made in other cultures, and it shows a way of reconciling the idea that we can have moral knowledge with the existence of apparently irresolvable differences in moral beliefs held in different cultures. Nevertheless, a number of strong philosophical objections to cultural relativism exist.

Objections to cultural relativism

PROBLEMS OF APPLICATION

To make sense of moral discourse in the way recommended by the cultural relativist, we need to be able to identify the culture to which the speaker belongs, and to verify the claim that some behaviour is or is not approved of in that culture. Both of these things will be difficult – even impossible – to do in many cases, especially in pluralist cultures like ours. How do we identify the culture to which an individual belongs? This can hardly be done simply by seeing what state they belong to, for there may be a number of quite radically different cultural groupings co-existing within the boundaries of the same state. Australia is often referred to as a multicultural society, and clearly there are important differences between the culture of outback Aborigines, and that of inner-city yuppies, for instance. Even *within* one of these groupings, there may be significant variations in attitude and behaviour: some yuppies engage in and approve of taking illegal drugs and some disapprove of it. Should each of these groups of yuppies be counted as different cultures? There seems no obviously correct method for resolving this question.

Furthermore, groups which we generally think of being part of the same culture often exhibit a range of attitudes to a particular kind of behaviour. Say we decide that we will count inner-city yuppies as belonging to one culture, and we ask if, for this group, taking illegal drugs is good. On the cultural relativist account this means that we are inquiring if this behaviour is approved of in the yuppies' culture. If it is, then it is good, and if it is not approved, then it is bad. But, as we have claimed, it is *both* approved and disapproved of in yuppie culture: on the relativist account this means that it is both good and bad at the same time. But what can it mean to call something both good and bad simultaneously? (Though something can be good in some respects and bad in other respects at the same time, this is not what is meant here.)

A good moral theory yields determinate answers to moral questions: questions about what is morally good and bad, what morally ought to be done and not done, and so on. Cultural relativism, however, would appear not always able to provide such answers. The cultural relativist is committed to the idea that the truth or falsity of a statement asserting that some behaviour is good is to be determined by seeing whether or not it is approved of in the agent's culture. But we have seen that (at least some of the time) there is no obvious way of deciding which culture the agent belongs to. Even where there is a way, often there is no clear answer to the question of whether the assertion is true or false.

PROBLEMS OF COMPREHENSIVENESS

Another desideratum for a good theory is that it be comprehensive, in the sense that it can explain and make sense of the whole range of phenomena which fall under its purview. A theory of weather would not be comprehensive if it had nothing to say about rain, for example. Cultural relativism seems to lack comprehensiveness.

In particular, cultural relativism seems unable to accommodate the idea of moral progress (or regression). To illustrate this, let us consider the practice of slavery, as it existed in America. In the 17th and 18th centuries slavery was generally approved of in American society; so on the cultural relativist approach slavery was good (for Americans). Nowadays, slavery is generally disapproved of in American society; so on the relativist approach slavery is now bad (for Americans). Most of us, of course, believe that the abolition of slavery was a morally good thing, and that in this respect American society became morally better when it happened. We think this because we believe that slavery was bad, for example because it treated people as chattels, so abolishing slavery constituted moral progress. But all the cultural relativist can say is that at one time slavery in America was good – because it was generally approved – and subsequently, when that approval was withdrawn, it became bad. There is simply no room in the theory to make the further claim that this change represented moral progress. So it seems unable to accommodate a significant part of the realm of moral discussion and judgment.

PROBLEMS OF MEANING

We saw above that cultural relativism rests on a claim about the meaning of moral terms. The cultural relativist thinks, for example that the term 'morally good' *means* 'approved of in the agent's society'. Let's look at this claim.

If one term means the same as another then they pick out just the same things in the world; moreover, whatever is true of this thing, given one way of referring to it, is true given the other way of referring to it. It's probably easiest to grasp this through the use of examples.

The word 'oculist' means the same as the words 'eye-doctor'; an oculist just is an eye-doctor. Consider the following sentence:

1) Most oculists are over 35.

If this sentence is true, then so is this one:

2) Most eye-doctors are over 35.

Sentence 2) doesn't simply *happen* to be true: given the truth of 1) and the equivalence of meaning between 'oculist' and 'eye-doctor' it *must* be true.

We *know* that the terms 'oculist' and 'eye-doctor' mean the same thing.

Sometimes, of course, claims about the equivalence of meaning are more controversial. It is certainly a matter of controversy that 'morally good' means 'approved of in the agent's society', as cultural relativists claim. The English philosopher GE Moore developed what he called 'The Open Question Argument' to point out the implausibility of the claims about the meaning of moral terms made by theories like cultural relativism. An open question is simply a question where the answer could be either positive or negative: yes or no. Moore pointed out that if two terms really mean the same thing then it cannot be an open question whether what is true of one of the terms is also true of the other (Moore 1903). So consider the question:

'Most oculists are over 35, but are most eye-doctors over 35?'

Given the meaning of the terms 'oculist' and 'eye-doctor' this is not an open question; the answer simply has to be 'yes'. (Indeed it is difficult to see what the point of asking such a question could be.)

Let's apply the open question test to the claims about the meaning of moral terms made by the cultural relativist.

Recall that the cultural relativist thinks that 'morally good' means 'approved of in the agent's society'. Now consider this question:

'Meat eating is generally approved of in our society, but is meat eating morally good?'

If the cultural relativist is correct about the meaning of moral terms, then this will not be an open question; since meat eating is approved in our society it *must* be true that it is morally good. But surely this question *is* an open question. After all, it is a matter of real moral controversy as to whether or not meat eating is morally acceptable, and it is at least conceivable that even though it is true that meat eating is approved, it is nevertheless wrong. This point can be generalised to apply to a whole range of socially-sanctioned activities in our own and other societies. The cultural relativist's claim about the meaning of moral terms does not stand up.

THE CLAIMS OF TOLERANCE

The theory of cultural relativism arose at least in part as an understandable reaction against the attitudes displayed to non-European ways of life by many Europeans. From the 18th century until well into the 20th these attitudes were informed by theories of culture, which claimed that a hierarchy of social development existed. These theories placed 'civilised' peoples (such as the British) at the top, and 'primitive' hunter-gatherers (such as Australian Aborigines) at the bottom. They thereby legitimised European colonists in forcing their own standards on the peoples they ruled, in the name of moral progress, in the process often destroying or radically reshaping indigenous cultures. The intolerant colonists, we now think, were wrong in imposing their moral standards on the peoples they colonised. But if the colonists were wrong, would we not be equally wrong – and equally intolerant – in judging the views and habits of other cultures in the light of our own moral standards?

The current attraction of cultural relativism rests to a large extent on such appeals to the value of tolerance. Tolerance properly understood, however, does not support cultural relativism. As we pointed out above, there is a general presumption that other people are morally autonomous, capable of responding to reasons, and freely choosing their actions. One of the implications of this presumption is that there is, as it were, a 'right to be wrong'. We have no right to interfere with other autonomous individuals' actions, unless they are hurting others. Tolerance, then, is a way of expressing our respect for autonomy. To accept others as morally autonomous is to see them as people to whom it is appropriate to respond to with, say, disapproval if they act badly, and praise if they act well. Conversely, we do not think that those who are lacking autonomy, such as very young children, or sufferers of senile dementia can or should be held morally responsible for their behaviour.

To think that we cannot, or must not, pass judgment on the behaviour of people from other cultures, then, far from exhibiting respect or tolerance, is actually implying that such people are not really morally autonomous agents at all. Of course, we should be cautious in making such judgments when we are dealing with cultures remote from our own, for as we saw above, ways of behaving that appear at first glance to be totally unacceptable, may look very different once we understand the values that they are expressing or the context in which they occur. But to say that we should be cautious in doing this, is very different from saying that we should not do it at all.

Finally, we should notice that the very values which make tolerance attractive, in some circumstances legitimate direct, coercive interference with other cultures. For instance, when the British colonised India, they discovered that the practice of burning widows on the funeral pyres of their dead husbands ('suttee') was widespread and culturally sanctioned. Such a practice involved the worst and most direct violation of the widows' autonomy. The British were justified in forcibly preventing it, by exactly the same considerations of autonomy as underpin the value of tolerance.

If cultural relativism were true we could act in the morally correct way by conforming to the norms of our society. We have seen a number of reasons to think that cultural relativism is not correct however. If it is not, then it seems unlikely that mere conformity will be sufficient to guide us to morally acceptable behaviour. Rather, in many cases we will have to reason about how to act. In the chapters that follow, we look firstly at the way we can reason about moral choices in general, then consider particular controversial issues to which such reasoning can be applied.

Readings

Benedict, Ruth (1934, 1968) *Patterns of Culture*, Routledge & Kegan Paul, London, pp 142–44.

— (1934) 'Culture and the abnormal', *Journal of General Psychology*, p 1.

Berndt, Ronald and Catherine (1992) *The World of the First Australians: Aboriginal Traditional Life: Past and Present*, Aboriginal Studies Press, Canberra, p 165.

Cicero, Marcus Tullius (1937) *In Catilinam II*, Lord, Louis E (translator), William Heinemann Ltd, London, pp 22–23.

Herodotus of Halicarnassus (1988) *The Histories*, Penguin, Harmondsworth, pp 219–20.

Joyce, Richard (2001) *The Myth of Morality*, Cambridge University Press, Cambridge.

Kellenberger, James (1979) 'Ethical relativism', *Journal of Value Inquiry*, vol 13, no 1, March, pp 1–20.

Levy, Neil (2002) *Moral Relativism*, Oneworld, Oxford.

Mackie, John (1977) *Ethics: Inventing Right and Wrong*, Penguin, New York.

Moore, George Edward (1903) *Principia Ethica*, available at <http://www.fair-use.org/g-e-moore/principia-ethica> (accessed 21/1/09).

Moser, Paul K and Carson, Thomas L (eds) (2001) *Moral Relativism: A Reader*, Oxford University Press, New York.

Turnbull, Colin (1972) *The Mountain People*, Simon & Schuster, New York, pp 135–36.

Williams, Bernard (1972) 'Interlude: Relativism' in Williams, Bernard (1972) *Morality: An Introduction to Ethics*, Harper & Row, New York.

Wong, David (1984) *Moral Relativity*, University of California Press, Berkeley.

3: Moral principles

[The following case study is taken from the novel Billy Budd. The setting is the British naval ship Bellipotent in 1797, following two notorious mutinies at Spithead and Nore. Billy Budd, a sailor on the Bellipotent, is gentle and trusting and well-loved by the crew. He is also uneducated and has trouble speaking when upset. John Claggart, Billy's superior officer, is a malicious and cruel man who deeply resents Billy's kindly nature and popularity among the men. Billy is unaware of Claggart's hatred until the moment he brings Billy before the ship's master, Captain Vere, and falsely accuses Billy of plotting a mutiny. Billy, stunned by Claggart's vicious lies, strikes out at him, accidentally killing him by the blow.

Captain Vere sets up a military tribunal. According to military law the penalty for striking a superior officer is death by hanging. After the evidence is heard and Budd cross-examined, Captain Vere addresses the court.]

What he said was to this effect: 'Hitherto I have been but the witness, little more; and I should hardly think now to take another tone, that of your coadjutor for the time, did I not perceive in you – at the crisis too – a troubled hesitancy, proceeding, I doubt not, from the clash of military duty with moral scruple – scruple vitalised by compassion. For the compassion, how can I otherwise than share it? But, mindful of paramount obligations, I strive against scruples that may tend to enervate decision. Not, gentlemen, that I hide from myself that the case is an exceptional one. Speculatively regarded, it well might be referred to a jury of casuists. But for us here, acting not as casuists or moralists, it is a case practical, and under martial law practically to be dealt with.'

'But your scruples: do they move as in a dusk? Challenge them. Make them advance and declare themselves. Come now; do they import something like this: If, mindless of palliating circumstances, we are bound to regard the death of the master-at-arms as the prisoner's deed, then does that deed constitute a capital crime whereof the penalty is a mortal one? But in natural justice is nothing but the prisoner's overt act to be considered? How can we adjudge to summary and shameful death a fellow creature innocent before God, and whom we feel to be so? Does that state it aright? You sign sad assent. Well, I too feel that, the full force of that. It is Nature. But do these buttons that we wear attest that our allegiance is to Nature? No, to the King. Though the ocean, which is inviolate Nature primeval, though this be the element where we move and have our being as sailors, yet as the King's officers lies our duty in a sphere correspondingly natural? So little is that true, that in receiving our commissions we in the most important regards ceased to be natural free agents. When war is declared are we the commissioned fighters previously consulted? We fight at command. If our judgements approve the war, that is but coincidence. So in other particulars. So now. For suppose condemnation to follow these present proceedings. Would it be so much we ourselves that would condemn as it would be martial law operating through us? For that law and the rigour of it, we are not responsible. Our vowed responsibility is in this: That however pitilessly that law may operate in any instances, we nevertheless adhere to it and administer it.

'But the exceptional in the matter moves the hearts within you. Even so too is mine moved. But let not warm hearts betray heads that should be cool. Ashore in a criminal case, will an upright judge allow himself off the bench to be waylaid by some tender kinswoman of the accused seeking to touch him with her tearful plea? Well, the heart here, sometimes the feminine in man, is as that piteous woman, and hard though it be, she must here be ruled out.'

He paused, earnestly studying them for a moment; then resumed.

'But something in your aspect seems to urge that it is not solely the heart that moves in you, but also the conscience, the private conscience. But tell me whether or not, occupying the position we do, private conscience should not yield to that imperial one formulated in the mode under which alone we officially proceed?' ...

In brief, Billy Budd was formally convicted and sentenced to be hung at the yardarm in the early morning watch, it now being night.

Herman Melville (1962) *Billy Budd: Sailor*

CASE STUDY 3.2

At another table near by, a student, who was unknown to him and whom he did not remember ever seeing, was sitting with a young officer. They were playing billiards and drinking tea. Suddenly he heard the student talking about the moneylender Alena Ivanovna ...

'She's quite famous', he said; 'she always has money to lay out. She's as rich as a Jew, she can put her hands on five thousand roubles at once, and yet she doesn't turn up her nose at the interest on a rouble. A lot of our fellows have been to her. But she's an old bitch ...'

And he began to recount how spiteful and cranky she was, and how, if payment was only one day overdue, the pledge would be lost. She would lend only a quarter as much as things were worth, she would demand five or even seven per cent a month, and so on. The student's tongue had run away with him, and, among other things, he informed his hearer that the old woman had a sister, Lizaveta, whom the vicious little thing was always beating and whom she kept in complete subjection and treated as if she were a child, although Lizaveta stood at least five foot ten ...

'Let me ask you a serious question', went on the student, even more heatedly. 'I was joking just now, of course, but look here: on the one hand you have a stupid, silly, utterly unimportant, vicious, sickly old woman, no good to anybody, but in fact quite the opposite, who doesn't know herself why she goes on living, and will probably die tomorrow without any assistance. Do you understand what I am saying?'

'Oh, I follow you', answered the officer, earnestly studying his companion's vehemence.

'Listen, then. On the other hand you have new, young forces running to waste for want of backing, and there are thousands of them, all over the place. A hundred, a thousand, good actions and promising beginnings might be forwarded and directed aright by the money that old woman destines for a monastery; hundreds, perhaps thousands, of existences might be set on the right path, scores of families saved from beggary, from decay, from ruin and corruption, from the lock hospitals – and all with her money! Kill her, take her money, on condition that you dedicate yourself with its help to the service of humanity and the common good: don't you think that thousands of good deeds will wipe out one little, insignificant transgression? For one life taken, thousands saved from corruption and decay! One death, and a hundred lives in exchange – why, it's simple arithmetic! What is the life of that stupid spiteful, consumptive old woman weighed against the common good? No more than the life of a louse or cockroach – less, indeed, because she is actively harmful.'

Fyodor Dostoevsky (1973) *Crime and Punishment*

CASE STUDY 3.3

In 1939 British Intelligence obtained through the Polish Secret Service a copy of the German cypher machine 'Enigma'. A team of cryptanalysts working at Bletchley Park succeeded in breaking the German codes and were thus able to supply the Allies with much advance information about Axis plans. As a result at 3 pm on 14 November 1940 the team at Bletchley Park intercepted a German signal which gave [Winston] Churchill at least 5 hours warning of the Coventry raid. FW Winterbotham, the man responsible for passing information from the 'most secret source' to Churchill saw the Prime Minister's dilemma like this:

> If Churchill decided to evacuate Coventry, the press, indeed everybody would know we had pre-knowledge of the raid and some counter-measure might be necessary to protect the source which would obviously become suspect.

... Churchill had to balance the lives that might be saved by evacuating Coventry against the lives that might be lost by endangering the source and thus cutting the Allies off from other information which might well shorten the war and save lives ... clearly, he was involved in sacrificing some lives so that others might be saved – not an uncommon experience in war.

John Harris (1980) *Violence and Responsibility*

CASE STUDY 3.4

Jim finds himself in the central square of a small South American town. Tied up against the wall are a row of twenty Indians, most terrified, a few defiant, in front of them several armed men in uniform. A heavy man in a sweat-stained khaki shirt turns out to be the captain in charge and, after a good deal of questioning of Jim which establishes that he got there by accident while on a botanical expedition, explains that the Indians are a random group of the inhabitants who, after recent acts of protest against the government, are just about to be killed to remind other possible protesters of the advantages of not protesting. However, since Jim is an honoured visitor from another land, the captain is happy to offer him a guest's privilege of killing one of the Indians himself. If Jim accepts, then as a special mark of the occasion, the other Indians will be let off. Of course, if Jim refuses, then there is no special occasion, and Pedro here will do what he was about to do when Jim arrived, and kill them all. Jim, with some desperate recollections of schoolboy fiction, wonders whether if he got hold of a gun, he could hold the captain, Pedro and the rest of the soldiers to threat, but it is quite clear from the set-up that nothing of the kind is going to work: any attempt at that sort of thing will mean that all the Indians will be killed, and himself. The men against the wall, and the other villagers, understand the situation, and are obviously begging him to accept. What should he do?

Bernard Williams (1980) 'A critique of utilitarianism'

CASE STUDY 3.5

Justifying her decision, the City Planner explained that there were only two possible routes for the freeway, either of which would have cost about the same.

'Either way we would have to have resumed some houses for destruction. But if we had gone through Olympic Heights we would have to have demolished over a hundred family homes. By taking the Parkdale route we only have to get rid of six.'

In response to a question the City Planner denied that any political pressure had been applied on behalf of the influential Parkdale residents to save their expensive homes. 'Even if there had been, it would have made no difference to me. In the circumstances all I considered was the numbers affected.'

Provided by the authors

CASE STUDY 3.6

I will refer to the case of a pupil of mine, who sought me out in the following circumstances. His father was quarrelling with his mother and was also inclined to be a 'collaborator'; his elder brother had been killed in the German offensive of 1940 and this young man, with a sentiment somewhat primitive but generous, burned to avenge him. His mother was living alone with him, deeply afflicted by the semi treason of his father and by the death of her eldest son, and her only consolation was in this young man. But he, at this moment, had the choice between going to England to join the Free French Forces or of staying near his mother and helping her to live. He fully realised that this woman lived only for him and that his disappearance or per- haps his death – would plunge her into despair.

Consequently, he found himself confronted by two very differ- ent modes of action; the one concrete, immediate, but directed towards only one individual; and the other an action addressed to an end infinitely greater, a national collectivity, but for that very reason ambiguous – and it might be frustrated on the way. At the same time, he was hesitating between two kinds of morality; on the one side the morality of sympathy, of personal devotion and, on the other side, a morality of wider scope but of more debatable validity. He had to choose between those two. What could help him to choose?

Which is the more useful aim, the general one of fighting in and for the whole community, or the precise aim of helping one particu- lar person to live? Who can give an answer to that *a priori*? No-one. Nor is it given in any ethical scripture. The Kantian ethic says, Never regard another as a means, but always as an end. Very well; if I remain with my mother, I shall be regarding her as the end and not as a means: but by the same token I am in danger of treating as means those who are fighting on my behalf; and the converse is also true, that if I go to the aid of the combatants I shall be treating them as the end at the risk of treating my mother as a means ...

In coming to me, he knew what advice I should give him, and I had but one reply to make. You are free, therefore choose – that is to say, invent. No rule of general morality can show you what you ought to do: no signs are vouchsafed in this world.

Jean-Paul Sartre (1948) *Existentialism and Humanism*

CASE STUDY 3.7

At 8:46 on the morning of September 11, 2001, the United States became a nation transformed.

An airliner travelling at hundreds of miles per hour and carrying some 10 000 gallons of jet fuel ploughed into the North Tower of the

World Trade Center in Lower Manhattan. At 9:03 a second airliner hit the South Tower. Fire and smoke billowed upward. Steel, glass, ash, and bodies fell below. The Twin Towers, where up to 50 000 people worked each day, both collapsed less than 90 minutes later.

At 9:37 that same morning, a third airliner slammed into the western face of the Pentagon. At 10.03, a fourth airliner crashed in a field in southern Pennsylvania. It had been aimed at the United States Capitol or the White House, and was forced down by heroic passengers armed with the knowledge that America was under attack.

More than 2600 people died at the World Trade Center; 125 died at the Pentagon; 256 died on the four planes. The death toll surpassed that at Pearl Harbor in December 1941.

This immeasurable pain was inflicted by 19 young Arabs acting at the behest of Islamist extremists headquartered in distant Afghanistan. Some had been in the United States for more than a year, mixing with the rest of the population. Though four had training as pilots, most were not well-educated. Most spoke English poorly, some hardly at all. In groups of four or five, carrying with them only small knives, box cutters, and cans of Mace or pepper spray, they had hijacked the four planes and turned them into deadly guided missiles.

The 9/11 Commission Report, Final Report of the National Commission on Terrorist Attacks Upon the United States (2004)

ETHICAL ANALYSIS

In our everyday decision-making we make use of general rules or principles. We apply these to a range of situations to help us to decide how to act. In our financial decision-making we follow rules or principles, such as 'Don't lend money to those we do not trust or who are unable to make repayments.' In our work we follow rules and principles, such as 'Wear hard hats on construction sites', 'Consult all interested parties before formulating the policy on the new freeway', and so on. More generally, we follow the principle to do things that are in our self-interest, unless there are strong moral prohibitions against doing those things. These prohibitions are themselves rules or principles. Thus when it comes to moral decision-making we have recourse to rules or principles such as, 'Do not tell lies', 'Do not kill innocent persons', 'Treat others as you would have them treat you', 'Do not prevent people from engaging in actions you disapprove of unless those actions will harm others', and so on.

Sometimes moral or ethical decision-making is quite easy. The relevant moral principles are obvious; they dictate a certain course of action, and this action is also in our self-interest. For example, if I find the lost key of my boss, Joan, on the street I should return it to her. Firstly, there is a moral principle to assist others if there is little or no cost to oneself. Secondly, by helping out my boss I will win her favour and this may well benefit me in the future.

At other times our self-interest may be inconsistent with our moral duty. For example, it might be our moral duty to report a fellow worker who is milking the till, but it may not be in our self-interest because the worker in question is offering money to us to keep quiet and the risks of getting caught are non-existent. Here it may be psychologically difficult for us to make the right decision; partly because it is not in our interest to do so. Nevertheless, the situation is not morally problematic: it is not difficult to work out what the morally correct course of action is, even though it may be difficult to actually do what one knows is right.

Sometimes, however, we find ourselves confronting situations that are morally problematic. Although we want to do what is right, we are not sure what the morally right course of action is. These are typically situations in which each of a number of mutually exclusive options has moral principles and considerations in favour of it. Some of these principles or considerations favour one course of action, others favour a second course of action, and may even tell against the first. Yet only one course of action is possible. In these kinds of situations we need to think carefully about the relevant moral principles and considerations, and whether we ought to give more weight to one principle rather than the others. The above case studies are examples of this kind. Each of these case studies apparently involves a number of competing moral rules, principles or considerations.

Consider case study 3.1 involving Billy Budd. Billy Budd is a good person who accidentally killed an evil person, his superior officer John Claggart. Billy intentionally struck Claggart in a fit of anger at Claggart's vicious and untrue accusation that he had plotted a mutiny. If Billy is convicted of striking and killing Claggart the military law of the time demands that he hang.

Let us try and disentangle some of the moral complexities, including moral principles, in play here. On the face of it the decision to hang Billy Budd appears to be unjustified. Billy Budd is a good person who in a fit of justified anger struck Claggart; Claggart being someone who was trying to do him great harm. Though Billy intentionally struck Claggart out of anger he did not intend to kill him. Further, the world is surely a better place without Claggart than it is with him. From this perspective for Billy Budd to hang seems at the very least grossly unjust.

Let's make explicit some of the moral principles relevant to this situation and see how they apply.

Firstly, let us consider principles which might be called upon to support the claim that Billy should not be punished, or at least that his punishment should not be severe:

1) The good should be allowed to live (Billy was a good person).
2) We should not inflict immoral punishments. (The death penalty is an immoral punishment and if Billy is found guilty of striking Claggart he will be hanged.)
3) One should not be held fully responsible for one's unintentional actions (Billy did not intend to kill Claggart).
4) If you try to kill someone without good reason then you forfeit your own right to life (Claggart was in effect trying to bring about the death of Billy, since the result of a conviction for mutiny would have been Billy's death).

5) Always act to maximise the greatest good for the greatest number (other things being equal the world is better off with Claggart dead and Billy alive).

On the other side we have the following considerations:

6) Intentionally acting in a way that endangers or leads to the death of a human being is morally wrong (Billy intentionally struck Claggart, thereby causing his death).
7) It is morally wrong to break the law (Billy broke the law by striking Claggart).
8) Attacking military authority in wartime is wrong, since it tends to undermine the war effort and put the lives of one's fellow soldiers, and ultimately one's fellow citizens, at risk (Billy's striking Claggart constituted such an assault).
9) Breaking the law – including in this case striking one's superior officer – is stupid, since it cannot help and will invariably worsen one's situation. (If Billy Budd had not struck Claggart, Billy probably would have been found innocent of plotting mutiny and Claggart would have been disciplined.)

The overall moral situation of the trial of Billy Budd is a life and death matter. Billy has killed Claggart, and Billy's own life is to be taken. The situation is complex in virtue of the various competing moral considerations elaborated above, but it is also compelling. This is because a central moral value, namely life, is at stake. The other case studies are also complex and compelling, albeit in different ways.

Consider case study 3.2. Here killing the moneylender, Alena Ivanovna, is being weighed against the benefits to various deserving people of distributing her money, and also the apparent moral rightness of ridding the world of someone who creates only misery for others. On the one hand murder is wrong, on the other hand bringing about good consequences is morally right.

Case studies 3.3 and 3.4 involve decisions apparently largely based on the calculation of consequences. As illustrated in case study 3.5, matters of public policy are often decided simply by weighing the consequences of the various feasible alternatives on those affected, with equal weight being given to the interests of each. No doubt in the case of the location of a freeway we would think that the interests of the rich and well-connected should not be given greater weight than the interests of others. Is this kind of exclusively consequential reasoning equally plausible in the situation described in case study 3.3, and if so does it support Winston Churchill's decision not to warn the residents of Coventry of the imminent air-raid? The consequences of Churchill failing to warn Coventry is that innocent lives will certainly be lost in the very near future. On the other hand if he does warn Coventry, as a consequence many more innocent lives will be probably be lost in the somewhat more distant future. On the face of it, on a purely consequentialist calculation, with the interests of each affected person being given equal weight, Churchill should keep silent. However, even on purely consequentialist grounds, there are reasons for thinking that this judgment may be over-hasty. After all, Churchill *knows* that innocent people will die in Coventry if he does not act immediately. It is in his power to save these people. On the other hand, it is at best *likely* that if he acts to save the people in Coventry this will lead to more deaths of so far unknown people in the future than if he had not so acted. For the Germans may discover that their codes are being broken anyway, or it might be possible to make the Germans believe that information about the raid was obtained in some other way.

The dilemma faced by Churchill is importantly different from one in which a democratically elected leader might be thought to be called upon to deliberately kill innocent citizens in order to save the lives of a much larger number of innocent civilians.

Consider, for example, a variation on case study 3.7. Imagine that the US Air Force has been called upon to shoot down a US domestic airplane to prevent it crashing into the World Trade Centre during the infamous al-Qaeda attack on 9/11 (Miller 2009, pp 126–29).

Here the alleged dilemma is whether intentionally to refrain from protecting the lives of the innocent many (those in the building and its surrounds) or intentionally to kill the innocent few passengers (relatively speaking) to protect the lives of the innocent many (and given the passengers were almost certain to be killed in any case). This particular example seems to us not to be a dilemma for presidents, senior security personnel and other government officials in their capacity as government officials. Governments, including liberal democratic governments, are not, and cannot be, legitimately authorised to (in effect) execute some of their own citizens in order to save the lives of other people (whether they be their own citizens or not); or indeed for any other 'larger' purpose. The reason for this is simply that the moral legitimacy of governments – liberal democratic governments in particular – derives in large part from, and crucially depends on, respecting the human rights of autonomous human persons considered individually, and not simply in aggregate. Put simply, individual citizens in liberal democratic societies have not relinquished their right to life to governments. The only conditions under which governments may take the lives of their citizens intentionally are ones in which the rights to life of the citizens in question have been suspended by virtue of their own rights violations, for example, if these citizens are unjustifiably attacking other citizens.

Even if the government officials of liberal democracies – and perhaps of any morally legitimate system of government – are not, and could not be, justifiably authorised to intentionally take the lives of their own innocent citizens, scenarios like the one just described give rise to acute moral dilemmas for any human agent who has the opportunity to intervene; generally, such human agents will be, in fact, senior political, military or police personnel. These and other like dilemmas have given rise to ongoing and detailed philosophical debates between consequentialists and deontologists.

We do not have space to review these debates in detail here. Nevertheless, we note that it is far from self-evident that any human being has the moral right or moral duty to deliberately kill one or more innocent human beings in order to save the lives of other innocent human beings. For, arguably, the only morally acceptable justification for one human being deliberately killing another is that the second is an attacker, a rights violator or is otherwise not innocent. In short, only one's own moral fault can justify the suspension or overriding or discounting of one's right to life.

Most people would agree that unjustifiably trying to kill someone constitutes sufficient grounds for the suspension or overriding of one's right to life; more generally, moral fault in some sense diminishes one's moral rights. However, the question is whether or not there could be a different kind of justification, namely, one based on aggregating the value of individual lives. Thus, so the argument might go, I am justified in killing one innocent person in order to save 100, because 100 lives are a hundred times more valuable than one life.

One historically important line of philosophical reasoning here is provided by Immanuel Kant. In company with common sense morality, Kant believed that a human being is intrinsically – as opposed to instrumentally – morally valuable, and of greater value than non-human animals and inanimate objects. However, Kant also held the view that the moral value of human beings is such that one human being is not equivalent in moral value to, and therefore not replaceable without loss of value by, another human being, as is the case with, say, a piece of jewellery that has a price of $100 and, therefore, can be exchanged without loss of monetary value for a $100 note (Kant 1998, pp 42–43). Accordingly, the moral value that attaches to one human being is, numerically speaking, incommensurable with the moral value that attaches to another human being; the moral value of one human being is neither numerically equivalent to the moral value of another human being, nor is it numerically greater or smaller. Accordingly, it is not true that 100 human beings are 100 times as valuable as one human being.

The upshot of this is that deliberately killing a few innocents in order to save the lives of many innocents is inherently morally problematic. It necessarily involves doing what is morally wrong, given the incommensurable and 'undiminished' moral value that attaches to the life of an innocent person. For deliberately killing one or more innocent persons is morally wrong, irrespective of whether it was done in order to save the life of one or more innocent persons. On the other hand, deliberately refraining from saving the life of one or more innocent persons is also morally wrong, irrespective of whether it was done in order to avoid the morally wrong action of deliberately killing some other innocent person or persons.

At this point it will no doubt be pointed out that, other things being equal, it is morally worse deliberately to kill someone (that is, to do something to them to cause them to die) than it is deliberately to refrain from saving them (to allow them to die). This is so. Moreover, this moral difference between doing and allowing provides a rational decision procedure where the choice to be made is between the same number of innocent lives. Other things being equal, if one must choose between deliberately killing one innocent person in order to allow a second to live, and simply allowing the second innocent person to die and (as a consequence) the first to live, one should choose the latter option.

On the other hand, the moral difference between doing and allowing does not provide an entirely satisfactory solution to the kinds of moral dilemma under consideration here. For although not killing and not saving anyone in these types of circumstances is – other things being equal – the morally preferable option, it is still morally wrong to refrain from saving an innocent human being; one has done evil, albeit a lesser evil.

Invoking the doing/allowing distinction does not settle the question as to whether the number of lives to be taken or saved is a morally relevant consideration. What if one's choice is between deliberately refraining from saving one innocent person and deliberately refraining from saving 100 innocent persons? Or, even harder, what if one's choice is between deliberately killing one person and deliberately killing 100 innocent persons? That is, one cannot choose not to deliberately kill anyone.

It is self-evident – at least to most of us – that the numbers of human beings to be taken or saved is a moral consideration. However, what we have said thus far is not necessarily inconsistent with this.

The incommensurability thesis should not be confused with the thesis that the moral value of one human being is equivalent to the sum of the moral value of all other human beings. Nor should it be confused with the thesis that each human being has absolute moral value (whatever Kant might have thought on this issue). Rather we simply need to make the point that the numbers do make *some* moral difference; since the loss of one morally valuable entity is a bad thing then, presumably, the loss of two is a worse thing. However, this does not commit us to any simple process of numerical quantification, such as that advocated in classical utilitarianism, in the resolution of the kind of moral problem before us; it is not as if all we have to do is start counting and let the numbers arrived at do the rest.

So let us now return to the aeroplane scenario. The upshot of our discussion is that it is by no means clear that a government official, or anyone else, would be morally justified in deliberately killing the smaller cohort of innocent airplane passengers in order to save the lives of the larger cohort of innocent occupants of the building. Firstly, as we saw above, such a decision is not one a government official qua government official could justifiably be authorised to make. Secondly, other things being equal, it is morally preferable to avoid deliberately killing an innocent person than it is deliberately to refrain from saving an innocent person (that is, other things being equal it is morally preferable to allow the plane to crash into the building and kill the occupants than it is deliberately to kill the passengers in the plane oneself). Thirdly, although other things are not equal, given the smaller number of airplane passengers and the fact that the numbers count for something, this is not decisive. For the number of airplane passengers relative to the number of occupants of the building does not enable us – consistent with the dictates of morality (that is, with the principle of the incommensurability of the moral value of a human being) – to quantify numerically the moral value of a live cohort of airplane passengers relative to the moral value of a live cohort of occupants of the building.

There may, of course, be other softer options in a scenario like this one, such as impeding the further progress of the domestic airplane by disabling one of its engines and, thereby, causing it to make a crash landing. Under these circumstances the terrorists might seek to ensure that the plane does not land safely, but rather crash it, killing all on board. However, this would be an outcome deliberately caused by the terrorists. Crucially, even if the option of disabling the plane's engine had this outcome, it would not involve the deliberate killing of the passengers in the domestic plane by the authorities, albeit it might involve putting the passengers' lives at risk.

Here we are implicitly invoking the intended/foreseen consequences distinction. We take it that whether one deliberately intended an outcome, as opposed to merely foreseeing it, can make a moral difference. It is surely morally preferable to refrain from shooting dead an innocent person, even though one knows that if one does so refrain, the innocent person will be shot dead by someone else. Indeed, to choose the first option would be murder; not so, to choose the second.

That said, we take it that if one did not intend but did foresee, or ought to have foreseen, a harmful outcome of one's action, then this makes a moral difference. Other things being equal, an action with a foreseen (or foreseeable) harmful outcome is morally worse than the same action with an unforeseen (or foreseeable) but identical harmful outcome.

Moreover, we also take it that unintended, unforeseen and unforeseeable harm caused by one's actions is, other things being equal, morally worse than identical harm not caused by anyone's actions. Indeed, arguably, the latter kind of harm is not even susceptible of *moral* evaluation.

In short, whether a harmful outcome was intended or not can make a moral difference; and one greater than whether or not this outcome was foreseen (or foreseeable). However, internal states, such as intentions and beliefs, are not the only kind of thing to make a moral difference. Whether or not harm was *caused* by a human action also does. Indeed, the primary object of moral evaluation is a (deliberately) intended outcome that was caused by that very intention; which is to say, a morally significant human action.

Notwithstanding the above, in some cases this conceptual distinction between intended and foreseen consequences makes no moral difference, since it cannot be applied to the circumstances in question. Consider the well-worn philosopher's example of a man who smashes the fly on a second man's head with a sledgehammer, and then insists that cracking the poor fellow's skull was not intended, but merely a foreseen consequence of his action of 'swatting' the fly. This is implausible, not because there is no general distinction between intentions and foreseen consequences, nor because when the distinction applies then it is morally irrelevant. Rather, what the 'fly-swatter' claims is implausible, because in this particular case the distinction does not have application; it is a case of *intending* to crack the man's skull, and not merely foreseeing it as an outcome. A real-life terrorist scenario in which the intending/foreseen consequences distinction does not have application is the killing of the Hamas official Salah Shahada carried out by the Israeli military in Gaza in 2002. It involved the bombing (using a one-ton bomb) of his house, killing 13 other Palestinians, including children. As with the 'fly-swatter', it would be implausible for the Israelis to claim that they did not intend to kill anyone in the house other than Salah Shahada, but rather only foresaw that they would do so.

Notwithstanding the above discussion, it may nevertheless be true that *many* matters of public policy should be decided by reference to the consequences of the various available courses of action, and that equal weight should be given to the interests of those affected (Goodin 1985). Neither of these demands appears so plausible when it comes to making decisions about many matters in a private capacity. Though we often give weight to the consequences of our actions, we also often look to other factors, such as the nature of the available actions themselves. And it often appears legitimate to give special weight to the interests of our intimates – friends and family – or even to our own interests. (These issues are discussed in more detail in the following two chapters.)

Finally, it is worth reflecting on the point that Jean-Paul Sartre makes in his discussion of his student's dilemma in case study 3.6. He is in effect pointing out that the individual cannot evade responsibility for their action by appealing to some moral principle, even where that principle is a sound one. Moral principles are unlike, say, the principles of arithmetic, which cannot come into conflict with each other. Since moral principles can and do conflict with each other, a choice must be made as to what weight should be given to them in concrete situations of moral action. Such a choice is itself a moral action, for which the chooser must be prepared to take responsibility.

Bernard Gert's substantive moral theory

While we have discussed various moral principles, and categorised them in a variety of ways, we have not offered a comprehensive list of all the moral principles. Such a list might seem necessarily to be an extremely long, and perhaps indeterminate, one. However, many apparent moral principles, such as 'Do not steal from your employer', are reducible to other more basic moral principles, such as 'Do not steal'. At any rate, here we have an important philosophical question: 'Is there a determinate and comprehensive list of moral principles, and if so, what is it?'

One influential contemporary philosopher who has attempted to provide such a list is Bernard Gert.

Gert sees morality as a social contrivance that is meant to serve a certain purpose:

> The point of morality is to lessen the suffering
> of those harms that all rational persons want to
> avoid: death, pain, disability, loss of freedom and
> loss of pleasure. (Gert 2004, p 4)

According to Gert, a system is in place that governs our actions and decisions in order to achieve that function: he calls this 'common morality'. This

> ... is a system that rational persons put forward as
> a public guide for the behaviour of everyone who
> can understand it and guide their behaviour by it,
> that is, moral agents. (Gert 2004, p 4)

All rational agents are supposed to understand the kinds of behaviour that common morality 'prohibits, requires, discourages, encourages, and allows'. The fundamental categorical distinction which Gert discerns within the system of 'common morality' is between what he calls 'the moral rules', and the 'moral ideals'. Both 'rules' and 'ideals' can be seen as moral principles, though they differ from each other in important ways, discussed further below.

The common feature of the rules is that they prohibit the causing of harm. According to Gert there are 10 moral rules, which fall into two groups. The rules in both groups instruct us not to act in ways which will cause the five basic harms rational persons want to avoid, death, pain, disability, loss of freedom, and loss of pleasure. The first five moral rules are:

- Do not kill.
- Do not cause pain.
- Do not disable.
- Do not deprive of freedom.
- Do not deprive of pleasure.

These rules prohibit those kinds of actions that *directly* cause these harms. The second five rules are:

- Do not deceive.
- Keep your promises.
- Do not cheat.
- Obey the law.
- Do your duty.

These rules prohibit those kinds of actions that *indirectly* cause the five basic harms.

Moral ideals are also directed towards the lessening of the suffering of harms. But while we follow the moral rules simply by not harming, we have to engage in positive action to conform to the moral ideals. 'The moral ideals encourage people to prevent or relieve the harms that the moral rules prohibit them from causing' (Gert 2004, p 17). A volunteer who nurses war victims is clearly exemplifying a moral ideal in Gert's sense. Gert claims that the 10 moral rules account for all actions that are morally prohibited and required. We are morally required to take (or refrain from taking) an action if, and only if, it falls under one of the moral rules. Actions in accordance with the moral ideals, on the other hand, are not morally required, though they are of course permissible, and indeed to be encouraged (Gert 2004, pp 15–17).

Without necessarily endorsing everything that Gert has to say about the distinction between what he calls rules and ideals, it seems clear that our ordinary moral thought does display some such distinction. While we think it admirable if people help each other, we do not generally think that they must do so, except perhaps where they can easily do so, and if they do not the other person will suffer serious harm. However, we do think that each ought not to harm others. However, even if we accept that there is some distinction of the kind Gert points to, we can still question the actual list of rules Gert provides as basic. Arguably Gert's list both omits some basic moral principles, and includes some that ought not to be included (Alexandra and Miller 2005).

Let us turn first to those moral rules that prohibit actions that would otherwise indirectly cause harm. Perhaps the two most obvious omissions from the list are 'Do not steal or damage other people's property' and 'Do not defraud'. Theft and fraud certainly indirectly harm people, notably by depriving them of resources they need to live and exercise their freedom. A third apparent omission is 'Do not defame'. Defamation is the undeserved harming of someone's reputation. Certainly, harming someone's reputation indirectly causes harm (for example, loss of economic opportunities and therefore resources to freely act). Arguably, harming a reputation is not in itself a bad thing, since the person's good reputation might not be deserved. However, undeserved destruction of a reputation appears to be bad in itself. So perhaps harming reputations ought to be regarded as a sixth basic harm alongside do not kill, disable, deprive of freedom or pleasure, and do not cause pain.

It might be thought that theft and/or fraud and/or defamation are reducible to one or more of the other moral rules, specifically the rules not to deceive, to keep one's promises and/or not to cheat. But if I openly walk into your house and remove your household appliances, you will know all that has happened and by whom; so there is no deception. In addition, I might not have promised not to take your goods; so there is no breach of promise. Finally, it is difficult to see in what sense, if any, I have cheated you. Certainly, theft of this kind is not akin to (say) insider trading. In the latter case, but not the former, there is a competitive market situation governed by rules, and insider trading is breaking one of those rules to give someone an unfair competitive advantage. So theft does not necessarily involve deceit, the breaking of any promise or cheating.

Now consider fraud. This necessarily involves deception. But fraud also involves taking a benefit from someone to which you are not entitled. Accordingly, fraud is not reducible to deception. Moreover, while some frauds involve breaking promises, many do not. Consider a fraudster who pretends to be a blind, rich, old woman's long lost son. The old lady gives him an expensive present: a Rolls-Royce. No promise has been made or broken. Nor has the fraudster broken some rule in a competitive context, and thereby gained an unfair advantage; it is not a case of cheating. So fraud does involve deceit, but it is also more than deceit. Moreover, fraud does not necessarily involve breaking a promise or cheating.

Finally, let us consider defamation. It might be thought that defamation necessarily involves deceit, but this seems to be false. If I make known some actual unsavoury, but essentially irrelevant episode in the distant past of a public figure, this may destroy his or her reputation, but undeservedly so. This is not deceit, but it is defamation. Moreover, as we saw with the case of fraud, the fact that defamation may involve deceit is not necessarily a reason for not morally proscribing it; since deception is not all or even the most important moral element in defamation. The most morally important element in defamation is reputation; defamation being the undeserved destruction or diminution of reputation. Not does defamation necessarily involve the causing of pain or embarrassment, since the defamed person may never discover that he or she has been defamed. Indeed, it might be impossible for them to find out; they might, for example, be dead. We argue thus that theft, fraud and defamation should be added to Gert's list of basic moral rules. We also think that Gert is wrong to include as a basic rule that we should obey the law. In our view there is a moral obligation to obey *specific* laws and *specific* legal systems, but only because those laws/legal systems embody the moral rules and/or achieve collective goods not otherwise obtainable. On this account legal systems or laws as such do not generate moral obligations, even presumptive moral obligations that can be overridden. So the obligation to obey the law is entirely unlike the obligation to keep one's promises. Other things being equal, making a promise creates a moral obligation. Naturally, some promises – such as a promise to kill innocent people – do not create obligations, and some promises that do create moral obligations can be overridden in certain circumstances. However, other things being equal, the fact that there is an extant legal system prescribing a particular set of acts and omissions does not entail an obligation to obey those laws; rather it all depends on the laws in question. Consider a totalitarian state of the kind described in George Orwell's *1984*. Surely there is no obligation to obey many of the laws in such a state, such as those forbidding free expression of opinions? We conclude that there is no fundamental moral rule to the effect that one ought to obey the law.

While the nature of the moral rules and ideals is clear enough in broad outline, it is worth briefly pointing to some of their complexities. Firstly, while the distinction between the rules and ideals generally follows the not harming/helping distinction, this is not without exception. Most of the time, we can conform to the rules simply by not doing anything. We conform to the rule against assault by not committing physical violence against others, and so on. It is true that generally we have to do something to keep promises, but we do not have to (that is, there is no rule to the effect that we should) make promises in the first place. However, there are occasions when the moral rules require us to help others, not simply refrain from harming them. Consider the following example. A healthy young woman, on her way to a social engagement, sees a toddler fall into a shallow pond. There is no-one else in the immediate vicinity. It would take a moment for the woman to wade into the pond and rescue the toddler from the danger of drowning. Nevertheless, because she does not want to soil her expensive new clothes, she walks away, leaving the child to its fate. It seems clear that the woman has broken a moral rule, not simply failed to live up to a moral ideal. After all, we will surely think that she deserves severe blame for failing to help the child. It seems, then, we accept that there is a rule to help others, especially when we can provide that help without undue cost to ourselves, and when failure to do so will lead to a severe harm to another person. (It is the existence of this duty to rescue, and its possible conflict with the rule that we should not harm others which generates the tension in the airplane case discussed above.)

Secondly, from the fact that we are not obliged to live up to moral ideals and we are obliged to conform to the moral rules, we should not conclude that a rule must always override an ideal if they come into conflict. Imagine a situation where your invalid pensioner neighbour asks you to mind her child while she goes to purchase a pair of shoes which is on sale at a much reduced price. You know that she has little money but loves stylish footwear. However, you have promised to meet some friends for a drink. You may be justified in such a case in breaking the promise (that is, breaking a moral rule) in order to do an act of kindness (that is, live up to a moral ideal). The general point here is that we should obey the moral rules unless there is a good reason not to. In some cases, at least, a good reason might be that there was a more weighty reason to act on a moral ideal.

Ethics and impartiality

As we saw in Chapter 1, both consequentialist and deontological theories of morality focus on the rightness and wrongness of actions, though they disagree about the feature of an action which accounts for its moral value. These theories share another similarity, in that they both advocate a principle of impartiality as constitutive of moral decision making. On these accounts the facts that you are my friend, employee or brother are morally irrelevant. I should no more give your interests greater weight in my moral reasoning because of these facts than I should give greater weight to the interest of the rich over the poor, or the handsome over the homely.

From the point of view of another kind of moral theory, namely, so-called virtue ethics (which we discuss further in the next chapter), these approaches over-emphasise the rightness or wrongness of individual actions, and give insufficient weight to the moral character of persons. Moreover, they tend to be fixated with the moral property of impartiality; everyone is counted as one, and everyone must be treated impartially (whether this be in accordance with a principle of maximising happiness or a principle of universalisability or both). However, individual human beings stand to one another in different kinds of moral relationships, and strict adherence to impartiality can distort these moral relationships.

Consider in this context case study 3.6. On the one hand is the deep personal moral obligation of the young man to his mother. She will be inconsolable if he goes; her life will cease to be liveable. The young man has a powerful moral obligation to one person in particular. This is not a moral obligation he has to other people. On the other hand there are the legitimate moral demands made on him by the community to contribute to the war against the Nazis. How can he in all conscience live at home in safety, while his fellow citizens risk their lives daily to combat the Nazi threat to the community? Accordingly, the young man is in a dilemma. On the one hand there is a powerful interpersonal moral obligation to a single person. On the other hand he has a general moral obligation to a large number of people, many of whom he does not even know. However, the point is that one could not even feel the force of this dilemma if one viewed one's mother and a stranger impartially. One has obligations to one's mother that one does not have to strangers. Treating one's mother and a stranger impartially – at least when it comes to providing care and attention

– would be morally absurd. That is why one can contemplate staying with one's mother even though one has obligations to a thousand, or even a hundred thousand or more strangers.

Case study 3.4 draws attention to another problematic moral consideration from the point of view of an ethic of impartiality. This is the moral consideration of Jim's integrity. Jim believes strongly in the moral principle of not intentionally and directly killing another human being. He could not live with himself if he violated this principle, since he would be a murderer.

Unfortunately, Jim has to decide between the life of one Indian and the lives of 20. At the level of impartial consideration of all the human lives at issue and of consequences this seems easy enough. Surely one ought to choose to preserve the lives of 20 over the life of one single person. However, the situation is not so simple.

For one thing, as we saw above, the value of one human life is incommensurable with the value of another human life; we cannot simply quantify the lives at risk, ascribing equal numerical value to each. For another thing, again as we saw above, there is a moral difference between doing and allowing; to kill someone is, other things being equal, morally worse than to allow someone to die.

Moreover, Jim will not be the person to kill the 20, if they are killed. Pedro will kill the 20, if they are killed. But Jim will be the one to kill the Indian, if one and only one Indian is to be killed. So he will definitely be a murderer of one person if he intentionally kills the innocent Indian. Accordingly, he will have violated one of his own deepest moral principles; he will be a murderer. On the other hand if he does not kill the one Indian, he will not be the murderer of the 20. Pedro will be the murderer. Perhaps Jim will be in some attenuated sense responsible for the deaths of the 20, in that he could have prevented their deaths. But at least he will not have violated his principle not to intentionally and directly kill another innocent human being. He will not be a murderer. Accordingly, it might be argued, Jim ought not to kill the Indian; rather he ought to preserve his integrity. Preserving his integrity overrides considerations of consequences. On the other hand, perhaps preserving his integrity at the expense of the lives of 20 people is mere moral self-indulgence. We will be considering the ethic of impartiality further in forthcoming chapters.

Readings

Alexandra, Andrew and Miller, Seumas (2005) 'Common morality and "institutionalising" ethics', *Australian Journal of Professional and Applied Ethics*, vol 7, no 1, pp 24–33.

Brandt, Richard Booker (1992) *Morality, Utilitarianism, and Rights*, Cambridge University Press, Cambridge.

Donagan, Alan (1977) *The Theory of Morality*, Chicago University Press, Chicago.

Dostoevsky, Fyodor (1973) *Crime and Punishment*, Penguin, Harmondsworth, pp 82–85.

Gert, Bernard (1998, 2005) *Morality: Its Nature and Justification*, Oxford University Press, New York.

—— (2004) *Common Morality: Deciding What to Do*, Oxford University Press, Oxford.

Goodin, Robert E (1985) *Protecting the Vulnerable*, University of Chicago Press, Chicago.

Harris, John (1980) *Violence and Responsibility*, Routledge & Kegan Paul, London, p 91.

Kant, Immanuel (1785, 1998) *Groundwork of the Metaphysics of Morals*, Gregor, Mary (translator and editor), Cambridge University Press, New York (any edition).

Lyons, David (1965) *The Forms and Limits of Utilitarianism*, Oxford University Press, Oxford.

Melville, Herman (1924, 1962) *Billy Budd: Sailor*, University of Chicago Press, Chicago, pp 109–10.

Miller, Seumas (2009) *Terrorism and Counter-Terrorism: Ethics and Liberal Democracy*, Blackwells, Oxford.

Nagel, Thomas (1974) 'War and massacre' in Nagel, Thomas, Cohen, Marshall, Brandt, Booker, Richard and Scanlon, Thomas (eds) (1974) *War and Moral Responsibility*, Princeton University Press, Princeton.

Nagel, Thomas et al (eds) (1974) *War and Moral Responsibility*.

Ross, William David (1930, 2002) *The Right and the Good*, Oxford University Press, New York.

Sartre, Jean-Paul (1948) *Existentialism and Humanism*, Methuen and Co, London, pp 35–38.

Smart, John Jamieson Carswe and Williams, Bernard (eds) (1973) *Utilitarianism: For and Against*, Cambridge University Press, Cambridge.

The 9/11 Commission Report, Final Report of the National Commission on Terrorist Attacks Upon the United States (2004), Executive Summary, available at <http://www.9-11commission.gov/report/911Report_Exec.pdf> (accessed 22/1/09).

Williams, Bernard (1980) 'A critique of utilitarianism' in Smart and Williams (eds) (1973) *Utilitarianism: For and Against*, pp 98–99.

4: Virtues and vices

Apart from the pain that he still felt, the thing that Dean disliked most about being in hospital was the boredom. So he was very happy to see his old friend Adam walk through the door at visiting time. They spent an hour deep in conversation. As Adam rose to leave Dean thanked him for the visit.

'Oh, not at all' replied Adam. 'As you know, I am a Kantian, and I regard it as a duty for close friends to visit each other.'

The next day, Bob appeared at visiting time. Dean had been pondering Adam's explanation for his visit, and recounted it to Bob.

'As for myself' Bob responded, 'I don't believe there is any such general duty. *I* came because I calculated that I could increase the sum of human happiness more by visiting you than in any other way.'

Charles came to visit the next day. 'And you Charles, what principle motivated you to come here?' queried Dean.

'Principle … principle? I don't know about principles. I just thought that you might be bored and lonely and looking for some company. It just seemed the right thing to do somehow. After all, I am your friend!'

Provided by the authors

The story goes that Paul Kruger, dining at Queen Victoria's table, picked up his finger bowl and innocently drank the rose water from it. The Queen, having noticed the Afrikaner-president's ill-mannered behaviour and the astonished looks of her other guests, instantly proceeded to drink from her own rose water. This compelled all the rest to follow suit. Kruger's act was uncivilized. The Queen showed tact. His conduct was embarrassing. Hers saved him from embarrassment.

David Heyd (1995) 'Tact: Sense, sensitivity, and virtue', *Inquiry*

One incident is particularly vivid to me. It concerns a birthday party that Fanshawe and I were invited to in the first or second grade … It was a Saturday afternoon in spring, and we walked to the party with another boy, a friend of ours named Dennis Walden. Dennis had a much harder life than either of us did: an alcoholic mother, an overworked father, innumerable brothers and sisters. I had been to the house two or three times – a great, dark ruin of a place – and I can remember being frightened by his mother, who made me think of a fairy tale witch. She would spend the whole day behind the closed door of her room, always in her bathrobe, her pale face a nightmare of wrinkles, poking her head out every now and then to scream something at the children. On the day of the party Fanshawe and I had been duly equipped with presents to give the birthday boy, all wrapped with coloured paper and tied with ribbons. Dennis, however, had nothing, and he felt bad about it. I can remember trying to console him with some empty phrase or other: it didn't matter, no-one really cared, in all the confusion it wouldn't be noticed. But Dennis did care, and that was what Fanshawe immediately understood. Without any explanation, he turned to Dennis and handed him his present. Here, he said, take this one – I'll tell them I left mine at home. My first reaction was to think that Dennis would resent the gesture, that he would feel insulted by Fanshawe's pity. But I was wrong. He hesitated for a moment, trying to absorb this sudden change of fortune, then nodded his head, as if acknowledging the wisdom of what Fanshawe had done. It was not an act of charity so much as an act of justice, and for that reason Dennis was able to accept it without humiliating himself. The one thing had been turned into the other. It was a piece of magic, a combination of off-handedness and total conviction, and I doubt that anyone but Fanshawe would have pulled it off.

After the party, I went back with Fanshawe to his house. His mother was there, sitting in the kitchen, and she asked us about the party and whether the birthday boy had liked the present she had bought for him. Before Fanshawe had a chance to say anything, I blurted out the story of what he had done. I had no intention of getting him into trouble, but it was impossible for me to keep it to myself. Fanshawe's gesture had opened up a whole new world for me: the way someone could enter the feelings of another and take them on so completely that his own were no longer important. It was the first truly moral act I had witnessed, and nothing else seemed worth talking about. Fanshawe's mother was not so enthusiastic, however. Yes, she said, that was a kind and generous thing to do, but it was also wrong. The present had cost her money, and by giving it away Fanshawe had in some sense stolen that money from her. On top of that Fanshawe had acted impolitely by showing up without a present – which reflected badly on her, since she was the one responsible for his actions. Fanshawe listened carefully to his mother and did not say a word. After she was finished, he still did not speak, and she asked him if he understood. Yes, he said, he understood. It probably would have ended there, but then, after a short pause, Fanshawe went on to say that he still thought he was right. It didn't matter to him how she felt: he would do the same thing again the next time.

Paul Auster (1987) *The New York Trilogy*

Agathocles, the Sicilian, not only from the status of a private citizen but from the lowest, most abject condition of life, rose to become king of Syracuse. At every stage of his career this man, the son of a potter, behaved like a criminal; nonetheless he accompanied his crimes with so much audacity and physical courage that when he joined the militia he rose through the ranks to become praetor of Syracuse. After he had been appointed to this position, he determined to make himself prince and to possess by force and without obligation to others what had been voluntarily conceded to him. He reached an understanding about this ambition of his with Hamilcar the Carthaginian, who was campaigning with his armies in Sicily. Then one morning he assembled the people and Senate of Syracuse, as if he meant to raise matters which affected the republic; and at a prearranged signal he had all the senators, along with the richest citizens, killed by his soldiers; and when they were dead he seized and held the government of that city, without encountering any other internal opposition.

So whoever studies that man's actions will discover little or nothing that can be attributed to fortune, inasmuch as he rose through the ranks of the militia, as I said, and his progress was attended by countless difficulties and dangers; that was how he won his principality, and he maintained his position with many audacious and dangerous enterprises. Yet it cannot be called virtue to kill fellow citizens, to betray friends, to be treacherous, pitiless, irreligious. These ways can win a prince power but not glory. One can draw attention to the virtue of Agathocles in confronting and surviving danger, and his courageous spirit in enduring and overcoming adversity, and it appears that he should not be judged inferior to any eminent commander; nonetheless, his brutal cruelty and inhumanity, his countless crimes, forbid his being honoured among eminent men. One cannot attribute to fortune or virtue what was accomplished by him without the help of either.

Niccolò Machiavelli (1513, 1981) *The Prince*

ETHICAL ANALYSIS

In the previous chapter we looked at some influential principles which, according to their proponents, we should use as guides when we wish to act morally. In recent years a number of philosophers have expressed dissatisfaction, not so much with the details of these principles, but rather with the whole approach which would place this kind of principle-driven decision making at the centre of moral life. They think that such an approach has lost sight of the importance of *character*: the kind of person we are. With this focus on character has come a renewed interest in the concepts of virtue and vice. Virtues and vices are relatively fixed dispositions to act in a good or evil way, to be on the one hand, kind, courageous, tactful, and on the other mean, cowardly and insensitive. The possession and exercise of these virtues and vices partially constitute our character, they help make us the kind of person that we are.

Case study 4.1 illustrates one of the reasons for this kind of reaction against principle-based theories of morality. If we consider the three visitors to the invalid Dean, we are likely to feel that Charles is the one who shows the most morally appropriate attitude to his friend, yet he is the only one of the three who is *not* acting in order to conform to a moral principle. There seems to be something missing in the motivations of Adam the Kantian and Bob the utilitarian. Their actions do not seem to be primarily motivated by their concern for *his* wellbeing, but rather by their desire that *they* act in the morally correct way. While such a desire is obviously commendable, the moral life of someone who is *only* motivated by it seems to be lacking in important respects. The person who is always calculating the best thing to do is incapable of the spontaneous and heart-felt sorts of actions which we often find admirable.

Moral principles give us rules by which to act. This has its advantages, since rules are things which can be made explicit and apply equally to everybody. But those theorists who have insisted on the importance of character have pointed out that given the range of situations we find ourselves in and the complexities of the individuals we deal with, there is often no rule which can be meaningfully applied. In these cases we need what might be called moral sensitivity, and this is not something which can be reduced to a matter of rules or calculation. This is well illustrated in case study 4.2, describing Queen Victoria's response to one of her guests, Paul Kruger, drinking the rose water in his finger bowl. If things proceed in their normal course the other diners will use *their* finger bowls to clean their fingers, and Kruger realising his gaffe in the royal presence will feel embarrassed. Victoria, in order to save him this embarrassment, drinks her own rose water, and the others follow suit. We may feel that Victoria acted well here – as the writer says she displayed tact, and prevented embarrassment – and clearly her intention was kindly. However there is no rule to the effect that when faced with this sort of situation, one should act as Victoria did. In as much as there is any rule governing the situation, presumably it is the rule of etiquette which says that finger bowls are for washing fingers, not for drinking from, and this is a rule which Victoria broke. Just as there was no rule guiding Victoria's action, so there was no requirement for her to act the way that she did. If she had not drunk the water from the finger bowl she would have done nothing for which she could have been reprimanded.

It is difficult, if not impossible, to come up with more than very general prescriptions for virtuous action for two reasons. Firstly, the range, complexity and continually changing nature of the sorts of situations where we may have to act morally mean that we will never be able to come up with comprehensive action-guiding rules. It would be absurd to conclude, on the basis of Queen Victoria's action, that whenever one guest drinks the water from the finger bowl, so should all the others, for instance. Sometimes, even if the water drinker did not know the purpose of finger bowls they would feel little or no embarrassment at discovering their mistake. Victoria's action was sagacious *in the circumstances*; in other circumstances it may be merely eccentric.

The second reason is connected to the first, but instead of focussing on the difference in circumstances, it looks to the difference in morally legitimate responses made by individuals to those circumstances. Tact is a virtue, but so is dignity, and if Queen Victoria had decided that drinking from a finger bowl would detract from her dignity, her decision not to do so would have been understandable and morally defensible. It was claimed above that the possession and exercise of virtues (and vices) help make us the kind of person we are. But just as circumstances display an inexhaustible variety, so do people. Two good people can differ in which virtues they place more emphasis on, which they are more likely to manifest, and hence on the responses they make to particular situations. Though their responses may be different, they might both be seen as reasonable, even commendable.

Case study 4.3 displays the way the virtues bear on the particularity of the situation a person finds themselves in. But it also shows how reasonable, morally sensitive people may differ in their interpretation of that situation. In order to help us appreciate the nature of Fanshawe's handing over his gift to Dennis, the narrator goes into considerable detail about Dennis's family situation, allowing us to understand why he would not have a gift, and why Fanshawe's handing over his gift is accepted and has the effect it does. To understand and judge Fanshawe's action we cannot simply see it as a case of one boy handing over his present to another boy who happens not to have one. We have to see it as a particular person giving his present to his friend, in the light of what he knows about how that person is likely to respond and the reasons for him not having a present. Fanshawe and the narrator think that Fanshawe did the right thing. Fanshawe's mother disagrees. It is not that she denies that Fanshawe displayed the virtue of generosity; rather she thinks that there were a number of overriding considerations which he did not sufficiently take into account. At least in part these considerations are couched in the language of virtue and vice: Fanshawe is accused of impoliteness (a minor vice) in turning up to the party without a present, and in being insufficiently sensitive to the effect that his actions had on his mother's reputation. Fanshawe, for his part, can also accept that his mother's concerns are legitimate, but for him they are not sufficiently weighty to convince him that he was wrong to act as he did. Through these differing responses we gain a keen insight into the difference in character of Fanshawe and his mother.

Characterising virtue

The discussion of virtue as central to the moral realm harks back at least to Aristotle, writing almost two and half thousand years ago. Modern theorists of virtue still have to take Aristotle's views seriously. In this chapter, though Aristotle will not be slavishly followed, most of the ideas are to be found in some form in his work *Nicomachean Ethics* (often referred to simply as *The Ethics*).

So far we have operated with an unanalysed notion of virtue and vice, taking it that courage, for example, is a virtue, in itself admirable, and cruelty a vice, to be despised.

As Aristotle pointed out, the term 'virtue' has a range of uses, not all which bear any moral implications. We can talk about the virtues of a knife, for instance: these include sharpness and ease of handling. We can similarly speak about the virtues of a clock, such as accuracy and quietness. Given that sharpness counts as a virtue in a knife, but not in a clock, what do these features of things have in common, such that they all can be called virtues? Each of them counts as a virtue because each helps the object in which they are found to achieve its function. The function of a knife is to cut: being sharp allows the knife to cut, so sharpness is a virtue in a knife. The function of a clock is to keep time: accuracy is necessary for it to be able to keep time, so accuracy is a virtue in a clock. Another way of talking about functions in this sense is to speak of ends: the end for which a knife is intended is cutting and so on. We are now in a position to offer a general characterisation of virtue. A virtue can be characterised as some property, the possession of which helps a thing achieve its end.

Human virtue

Such a characterisation of virtue may look quite unexceptionable when applied to artefacts, which have very clear functions. But what about human beings? Firstly, let's tentatively adjust the characterisation to fit more closely the notion of virtue as it applies to humans. (We'll make it more precise later.) A human virtue is some relatively stable aspect of someone's character which disposes the person to act in a way which will help them achieve their end. This characterisation begs the question: 'Can it be said that *we* have ends?' Well, sometimes at least, we clearly do, when we occupy certain roles. The function of a doctor is to cure the sick, a comedian's function is to make people laugh and so on. It is usually relatively simple to decide what are the various role virtues: courage in a soldier, diagnostic skill in a doctor, and so on; the qualities which help role holders achieve the ends of their role. We will look at these issues in more detail in Chapter 6. However, though it may be clear enough what the ends of people in their various roles are supposed to be, and hence what the relevant virtues are, it seems much harder to determine what the ends of human beings simply *as* human beings are; or indeed if they have any ultimate end at all. Aristotle thought that just as there is a final end, a highest good, of say medicine, which provided the standard for judging a doctor's work, so there is a final end which we possess just as people and against which we can judge human behaviour and institutions.

Aristotle was quick to acknowledge that there is a whole variety of particular goods which people actually aim at – at money, honour, friendship and so on – and which seem to have virtually nothing in common. Nevertheless, we can set up a kind of hierarchy among these goods. We can understand a good's place in this hierarchy in terms of means and ends. At the bottom of the hierarchy are those things which we value *only* as a means to some other end. So money is a good of this kind, since it has no intrinsic worth, it is valuable only in that it allows us to get other things which we value. (Some people – misers – do value money for its own sake, but they are simply making a mistake.) Next in the hierarchy come the things which we value not simply as means to ends, but also as ends in themselves, such as friendship, honour and pleasure. However, even these goods, though ends in themselves, are at the same time means to a further, and in Aristotle's view, final end. This end, at the top of the hierarchy, he calls *eudaimonia*. There is no exact equivalent for this term in English. It is often translated as 'happiness', but probably 'flourishing' is closer to Aristotle's meaning. This is the only good which is purely an end in itself. In the light of this good we can assess aspects of our characters to decide if they are virtues or not. Do they, could they, help us flourish? If they do, they will count as virtues, if they don't they won't.

By itself, being told that those aspects of our character which help us flourish count as virtues is not going to help us much, until we know what constitutes flourishing. Aristotle identifies flourishing strongly with the development and exercise of reason, which he takes to be the defining human property. We can, however, work with a less restrictive notion of flourishing. Some controversy exists about whether certain kinds of lifestyles and behaviours count as flourishing or not. While some people think of the life of silence of Trappist monks as a kind of spiritual mutilation, others think of it as offering sublime rewards. But at the same time often it is very clear if someone's life can be counted as flourishing. Someone who lives in pleasant surroundings, enjoying the company of congenial friends, doing interesting work, surely counts as having a flourishing life. And someone who lives in poverty and loneliness in a dangerous slum, does not have a flourishing life.

Consider the extract from Machiavelli's The Prince, case study 4.4, describing the career of the Sicilian tyrant Agathocles, who rose to a position of great power from very humble beginnings. To achieve this Agathocles displayed great perseverance, skill, courage and boldness. Normally, of course, we count these as virtues and admire the person who displays them. But how can we do either of these things in the case of Agathocles, since they were in the service of overweening ambition and allied to callous cruelty, treachery and disloyalty? If we take it that even though Agathocles was truly courageous, for example, but deny that in this case courage should be counted as a virtue, we are seemingly forced to accept the conclusion that the same sort of behaviour may sometimes count as virtuous and sometimes as vicious. How are we to make such judgments? One approach, deriving from Aristotle, is to appeal to the notion of 'the unity of the virtues' (Aristotle 1973, Bk 6, p 13). This means each of the virtues requires the others: it is impossible to be truly kind without being compassionate; to be truly brave without being fair, and so on. Above all one needs the kind of good judgment that allows one to act as required, to exercise one's virtues in the appropriate way: such judgment can be seen as a kind of executive virtue, marshalling the other virtues as required. Agathocles manifestly lacks many of the most important virtues (for instance, justice, compassion); to this extent he is morally deficient. Further, Agathocles' lack of important virtues prevents him from being able to exercise good judgment: Agathocles is deficient in the executive virtue. An important consequence of this inability of Agathocles to exercise good judgment – and, relatedly, of his lack of most of the important virtues – is that he cannot achieve a flourishing life, his worldly success notwithstanding. Thus, by Aristotle's lights, since Agathocles' courage is not contributing to his achieving a good life, it does not count as a virtue.

Developing virtue

A much broader range of behaviour is determined by instinct in other animals than it is in humans. In some ways the possession of instincts that guide behaviour is highly advantageous. Firstly, instincts are 'hard-wired', they are innate and develop irrespective of external stimuli; we have to learn how to build a house, spiders don't have to learn how to spin a web. Secondly, following from the first point, instinctual behaviour is automatic, there is no need for choice, calculation or judgment. For the range of our behaviour which is not guided by instinct we have neither of these advantages. Capacities to behave have to be developed, and their development depends on a whole range of contingent factors, such as the willingness of others to educate us. And we do need to choose, to calculate and to judge. In short, we have freedom in a range of areas. There are drawbacks to this freedom, but there are also advantages; it gives a greater flexibility and ability to innovate, for instance.

One area in which we have freedom is in the way we respond to our passions. Aristotle gives a neat list and characterisation of the passions: 'appetite, fear, confidence, anger, envy, joy, friendly feeling, hatred, longing, emulation, pity and in general the feelings that are accompanied by pleasure and pain' (Aristotle 1973, Bk 2, p 5). These feelings can pull us in opposite directions. I might be tempted to take the drink my host is offering because I am attracted by the pleasure which I will gain from it, but at the same time fear that if I do I will suffer in the morning. As we saw above, it is plausible that at least a lot of the time there is no formula we can appeal to in order to see what we should do. Even so, according to Aristotle, we can be certain that the right response will fall into a range, which he calls 'the mean': 'neither too much or too little' (Aristotle 1973, Bk 2, p 6). This distinction is often marked in our language. In the case of willingness to face danger, for instance, we have the mean of courage, flanked by cowardice (too little) and foolhardiness (too much). In our example of deciding whether to take the proffered drink we have the mean of temperance – taking sensual pleasure without overdoing it – flanked by licentiousness and wowserishness.

Again, to be told that we should aim for the mean may not seem very helpful unless we know what the mean is, and as we have seen, Aristotle and other virtue theorists deny that there is any formula or rule which can guide us here. Nevertheless, according to Aristotle, we can develop certain fixed states of character, dispositions to act, such that we will tend to make the right kinds of choices. Indeed, he thinks that in a morally mature person, once these dispositions have been developed, there will usually be no experience of conflict: acting virtuously will be seen and found attractive in itself.

To see the point here it might be helpful to distinguish between goods that are *extrinsic* and *intrinsic* to activities. Extrinsic goods are those that can be achieved *through* (or *by*) engaging in an activity, where that activity is instrumental to the achievement of the goal. For example, typically we engage in house cleaning in order to achieve the good of having a clean house. If houses did not get dusty and dirty, we would have no further reason to engage in house cleaning. Intrinsic goods, on the other hand, are goods that we get *in* engaging in some activity. So, we typically engage in recreational activities for their intrinsic goods. We play chess because of the pleasure to be had in playing chess. Likewise, when a good person acts in accordance with the virtues he or she thereby derives pleasure; the distinctive pleasure attached to being virtuous.

Certain states of character governing choice, then, can be identified as the virtues. These are the states that dispose us to act in a way that will be conducive to human flourishing. A virtuous *person* is one who finds the exercise of the virtues pleasant in themselves. A good *act*, correspondingly, is not simply one where the right choice is made, but one in which this choice is made for its own sake, not for some ulterior motive, and which arises out of the right kind of state of character.

Not everyone has the virtues in any significant degree, and everyone lacks them more or less totally in their first years. Given that the states of character that constitute virtue don't arise naturally and inevitably, how are they produced? Probably most importantly by habituation; we become a virtuous person by engaging in virtuous actions. On this view, moral education is fundamentally practical. Just as we become a swimmer by swimming, or a flute player by playing the flute, we become a good person by doing good things, by making the right choices. As Aristotle puts it: 'Neither by nature, then, nor contrary to nature do the virtues arise in us; rather we are adapted by nature to receive them; and are made perfect by habit' (Aristotle 1973, Bk 2, p 1). The process of choosing actions that the immature, imperfectly virtuous person must go through in their formative years, then, is both difficult and dangerous. Difficult, because they cannot yet have the developed character which tends to issue in the right choice; and dangerous because if a person consistently makes the wrong choice, they are likely to become habituated towards the extremes of behaviour rather than in the direction of the mean.

To *become* moral, on this picture, we need a moral education, practical guidance in choice. The process of learning to become moral can be compared to the process of becoming a competent speaker of our native language. Originally, we're likely to go wrong in all sorts of ways; we're put right by those who are already competent. At a certain stage, however, we become autonomous users of language. By this stage our linguistic habits, good or bad, are likely to be pretty well fixed. Similarly with moral behaviour. We can push this comparison between language use and morality further. Our use of language is creative: we are constantly using it in new ways, putting together strings of words that may have never been combined before, or at least not in our hearing. Such creativity is necessary if the language user is to be able to respond linguistically to the ever-changing nature of their world. Similarly, it might be claimed, the virtuous person needs to be able to respond appropriately to the constantly changing and varied situations of choice they find themselves in. And just as the competent speaker of a language is the standard of correctness in that language, so the virtuous person is the standard for correctness in moral action.

The virtuous community

In order for someone to gain the virtues, and thus have any hope of enjoying a flourishing life, they clearly have to belong to a certain sort of community, one in which they will be guided in the right sort of way. In other words, it is only within a community that is already largely virtuous that there is any hope of someone becoming virtuous. In turn, a community is unlikely to thrive for any length of time unless it is made up of virtuous people. So our nature demands that we live in a community, and that this community is properly organised; this is at least part of what Aristotle meant by his famous claim that 'man is a political animal'.

Since the internal arrangements and conditions in which communities live vary so much the virtues which are most important and the way in which the virtues are expressed will inevitably vary considerably from society to society. Virtue theory explains this variation, in fact uses it to support the claim that one of the advantages of becoming virtuous is the ability to deal with situations in their particularity.

Readings

Adams, Robert Merihew (2006) *A Theory of Virtue*, Oxford University Press, New York.

Aristotle (1973) *Nicomachean Ethics*, Thomson, James Alexander Kerr (translator), Penguin, Harmondsworth.

Auster, Paul (1987) *The New York Trilogy*, Faber and Faber, London, pp 210–12.

Baier, Kurt (1982) 'Virtue ethics', *Philosophic Exchange*, vol 3, Summer, pp 57–70.

—— (1988) 'Radical virtue ethics', *Midwest Studies in Philosophy*, vol 13, pp 126–35.

Becker, Lawrence (1975) 'The neglect of virtue', *Ethics*, vol 85, no 2, January, pp 110–22.

Darwall, Stephen (ed) (2003) *Virtue Ethics*, Blackwell, Oxford.

Dent, Nicholas (1984) *The Moral Psychology of the Virtues*, Cambridge University Press, Cambridge.

Flemming, Arthur (1980) 'Reviving the virtues', *Ethics*, vol 90, no 4, July, pp 587–95.

Foot, Philippa (1978) *Virtues and Vices and Other Essays in Moral Philosophy*, University of California Press, Berkeley.

Heyd, David (1995) 'Tact: Sense, sensitivity, and virtue', *Inquiry*, no 38, pp 217–31.

Hudson, Stephen (1980) 'Character traits and desires', *Ethics*, vol 90, no 4, July, pp 539–49.

Hurka, Thomas (2001) *Virtue, Vice, and Value*, Oxford University Press, Oxford.

Hursthouse, Rosalind (1999) *On Virtue Ethics*, Oxford University Press, Oxford.

Machiavelli, Niccolò (1513, 1981) *The Prince*, Penguin, Harmondsworth, Ch VIII, p 63.

MacIntyre, Alasdair (1981) *After Virtue*, Duckworth, London.

Sherman, Nancy (1989) *The Fabric of Character: Aristotle's Theory of Virtue*, Oxford University Press, Oxford.

Wallace, James (1978) *Virtues and Vices*, Cornell University Press, Ithaca NY.

Warnock, Geoffrey James (1971) *The Object of Morality*, Methuen, London, Ch 9.

5: Moral emotion, motivation and reasoning

A certain man went down from Jerusalem to Jericho, and fell among thieves, which stripped him of his raiment, and wounded him, and departed, leaving him half dead.

And by chance there came down a certain priest that way; and when he saw him, he passed by on the other side.

And likewise a Levite, when he was at the place, came and looked on him, and passed by on the other side.

But a certain Samaritan, as he journeyed, came where he was; and when he saw him he had compassion on him.

And went to him, and bound up his wounds, pouring in oil and wine, and set him on his own beast, and brought him to an inn, and took care of him.

And on the morrow, when he departed, he took out two pence, and gave them to the host, and said unto him, 'Take care of him; and whatsoever thou spendest more, when I come again, I will repay thee.'

Luke 10:30–35

On the night of March 13–14, 1964 thirty-eight New Yorkers were awakened in the early hours of the morning by the frenzied cries for help of a young woman, Kitty Genovese, the victim of a savage physical assault perpetrated by a man who had accosted her while she was on her way home. Over a period of about forty minutes, the assailant made several separate attacks on her, while she struggled, battered and bleeding, to reach the sanctuary of her apartment. Her screams of anguish and her calls for help were heard by at least thirty-eight neighbours, who, in the privacy and anonymity of their own homes, witnessed her struggle, yet offered no assistance in any form, whether through direct intervention or through the simple expedient of telephoning the police. A neighbour finally summoned the police, after first calling a friend to seek advice as to what to do. A patrol car arrived on the scene within two minutes but this prompt assistance was too late to save the young woman, who died on the way to hospital. It is clear that Kitty Genovese was a victim not only of her assailant's viciousness, but also of her neighbours' inaction.

Leon Shaskolsky Sehleff (1978) *The Bystander; Behaviour, Law, Ethics*

But, alas, I have not said all that I have to say about my time at Mme de Vercellis's. For though my condition was apparently unchanged I did not leave her house as I had entered it. I took away with me lasting memories of a crime and the unbearable weight of a remorse which even after forty years, still burdens my conscience. In fact the bitter memory of it, far from fading, grows more painful with the years. Who would suppose that a child's wickedness could have such cruel results? It is for these only too probable consequences that I can find no consolation. I may have ruined a nice, honest, and decent girl, who was certainly worth a great deal more than I, and doomed her to disgrace and misery.

It is almost inevitable that the breaking up of an establishment should cause some confusion in the house, and that various things should be mislaid. But so honest were the servants and so vigilant were M. and Mme Lorenzi that nothing was found missing when the inventory was taken. Only Mlle Pontal lost a little pink and silver ribbon, which was quite old. Plenty of better things were within my reach, but this ribbon alone tempted me. I stole it, and as I hardly troubled to conceal it was soon found. They inquired how I had got hold of it. I grew confused, stammered, and finally said with a blush that it was Marion who had given it to me. Marion was a young girl from the Maurienne whom Mme de Vercellis had taken as her cook when she had ceased to give dinners and had discharged her chef, since she had more need of good soup than of fine stews. Marion was not only pretty. She had that fresh complexion that one never finds except in the mountains, and such a sweet and modest air that one had only to see her to love her. What is more she was a good girl, sensible and absolutely trustworthy. They were extremely surprised when I mentioned her name. But they had no less confidence in me than in her, and decided that it was important to find which of us was a thief. She was sent for, to face a considerable number of people, including the Comte de la Roque himself. When she came she was shown the ribbon. I boldly accused her. She was confused, did not utter a word, and threw me a glance that would have disarmed the devil, but my cruel heart resisted. In the end she firmly denied the theft. But she did not get indignant. She merely turned to me, and begged me to remember myself and not disgrace an innocent girl who had never done me any harm. But, with infernal impudence, I repeated my accusation, and declared to her face that she had given me the ribbon. The poor girl started to cry, but all she said to me was, 'Oh, Rousseau, I thought you were a good fellow. You make me very sad, but I should not like to be in your place.' That is all. She continued to defend herself with equal firmness and sincerity, but never allowed herself any reproaches against me. This moderation, contrasted with my decided tone, prejudiced her case. It did not seem natural to suppose such diabolical audacity on one side and such angelic sweetness on the other. They seemed unable to come to a definite decision, but they were prepossessed in my favour. In the confusion of the moment they had not time to get to the bottom of the business; and the Comte de la Roque, in dismissing us both, contented himself with saying that the guilty one's conscience would amply avenge the innocent. His prediction was not wide of the mark. Not a day passes on which it is not fulfilled.

I do not know what happened to the victim of my calumny, but she cannot possibly have found it easy to get a good situation after that. The imputation against her honour was cruel in every respect. The theft was only a trifle, but after all, it was a theft and, what is worse, had been committed in order to lead a boy astray. Theft, lying, and obstinacy – what hope was there for a girl in whom so many vices were combined? I do not even consider misery and friendlessness the worst dangers to which she was exposed. Who can tell to what extremes the depressed feeling of injured innocence might have carried her at her age? And if my remorse at having perhaps made her unhappy is unbearable, what can be said of my grief at perhaps having made her worse than myself?

This cruel memory troubles me at times and so disturbs me that in my sleepless hours I see this poor girl coming to reproach me for my crime, as if I had committed it only yesterday. So long as I have lived in peace it has tortured me less, but in the midst of a stormy life it deprives me of that sweet consolation which the innocent feel under persecution. It brings home to me indeed what I think I have written in one of my books, that remorse sleeps while fate is kind but grows sharp in adversity. Nevertheless I have never been able to bring myself to relieve my heart by revealing this in private to a friend. Not with the most intimate friend, not even with Mme de Warens, has this been possible. The most that I could do was to confess that I had a terrible deed on my conscience, but I have never said in what it consisted. The burden, therefore, has rested till this day on my conscience without any relief; and I can affirm that the desire to some extent to rid myself of it has greatly contributed to my resolution of writing these *Confessions*.

I have been absolutely frank in the account I have just given, and no-one will accuse me, I am certain, of palliating the heinousness of my offence. But I should not fulfil the aim of this book if I did not at the same time reveal my inner feelings and hesitated to put up such excuses for myself as I honestly could. Never was deliberate wickedness further from my intention than at that cruel moment. When I accused that poor girl, it is strange but true that my friendship for her was the cause. She was present in my thoughts, and I threw the blame on the first person who occurred to me. I accused her of having done what I intended to do myself. I said that she had given the ribbon to me because I meant to give it to her. When afterwards I saw her in the flesh my heart was torn. But the presence of all those people prevailed over my repentance. I was not much afraid of punishment, I was only afraid of disgrace. But that I feared more than death, more than crime, more than anything in the world. I should have rejoiced if the earth had swallowed me up and stifled me in the abyss. But my invincible sense of shame prevailed over everything. It was my shame that made me impudent, and the more wickedly I behaved the bolder my fear of confession made me. I saw nothing but the horror of being found out, of being publicly proclaimed, to my face, as a thief, a liar, and a slanderer. Utter confusion robbed me of all other feeling. If I had been allowed time to come to my senses, I should most certainly have admitted everything. If M. de la Roque had taken me aside and said: 'Do not ruin that poor girl. If you are guilty tell me so', I should immediately have thrown myself at his feet, I am perfectly sure. But all they did was to frighten me, when what I needed was encouragement. My age also should be taken into account. I was scarcely more than a child. Indeed I still was one. In youth real crimes are even more reprehensible than in riper years; but what is no more than weakness is much less blameworthy, and *really my crime amounted to no more than weakness.* So the memory tortures me less on account of the crime itself than because of its possible evil consequences. But I have derived some benefit from the terrible impression left with me by the sole offence I have committed. For it has secured me for the rest of my life against any act that might prove criminal in its results. I think also that my loathing of untruth derives to a large extent from my having told that one wicked lie. If this is a crime that can be expiated, as I venture to believe, it must have been atoned for by all the misfortunes that have crowded the end of my life, by forty years of honest and upright behaviour under difficult circumstances. Poor Marion finds so many avengers in this world that, however great my offence against her may have been, I have little fear of carrying the sin on my conscience at death. That is all I have to say on the subject. May I never have to speak of it again.

Jean-Jacques Rousseau (1953) The Confessions

CASE STUDY 5.4

Surely, Lord, your law punishes theft, as does that law written on the hearts of men, which not even iniquity itself blots out. What thief puts up with another thief with a calm mind? Not even a rich thief will pardon one who steals from him because of want. But I willed to commit theft, and I did so, not because I was driven to it by any need, unless it were by poverty of justice, and dislike of it, and by a glut of evildoing. For I stole a thing of which I had plenty of my own and of much better quality. Nor did I wish to enjoy that thing which I desired to gain by theft, but rather to enjoy the actual theft and the sin of theft.

In a garden nearby to our vineyard there was a pear tree, loaded with fruit that was desirable neither in appearance nor in taste. Late one night – to which hour, according to our pestilential custom, we had kept our street games – a group of very bad youngsters set out to shake down and rob this tree. We took great loads of fruit from it, not for our own eating, but rather to throw it to the pigs; even if we did eat a little of it, we did this to do what pleased us for the reason that it was forbidden ...

When there is discussion concerning a crime and why it was committed, it is usually held that there appeared possibility that the appetites would obtain some of these goods, which we have termed lower, or there was fear of losing them. These things are beautiful and fitting, but in comparison with the higher goods, which bring happiness, they are mean and base. A man commits murder: why did he do so? He coveted his victim's wife or his property; or he wanted to rob him to get money to live on; or he feared to be deprived of some such thing by the other; or he had been injured, and burned for revenge. Would anyone commit murder without reason and out of delight in murder itself? Who can believe such a thing? Of a certain senseless and utterly cruel man it was said that he was evil and cruel without reason. Nevertheless, a reason has been given, for he himself said, 'I don't want to let my hand or will get out of practice through disuse.' Why did he want that? Why so? It was to the end that after he had seized the city by the practice of crime, he would attain to honours, power, and wealth, and be free from fear of the law and from trouble due to lack of wealth or from a guilty conscience. Therefore, not even Catiline himself loved his crimes, but something else, for sake of which he committed them.

Augustine (1963) *The Confessions of St Augustine*

CASE STUDY 5.5

Act 3 Scene I ...

ANTONY
Post back with speed and tell him what hath chanced:
Here is a mourning Rome, a dangerous Rome,
No Rome of safety for Octavius yet;
Hie hence and tell him so. Yet, stay a while;
Thou shalt not back till I have borne this corse
Into the market-place: There shall I try
In my oration how the people take
The cruel issue of these bloody men;
According to the which, thou shalt discourse
To young Octavius of the state of things.
Lend me your hand.
Exeunt [with Caesar's body].

Act 3 Scene 2

Enter Brutus and [presently] goes into the pulpit, and Cassius, with the Plebeians.

PLEBEIANS
We will be satisfied! Let us be satisfied!

BRUTUS
Then follow me and give me audience, friend.
Cassius, go you into the other street
And part the numbers.
Those that will hear me speak, let 'em stay here;
Those that will follow Cassius, go with him;
And public reasons shall be rendered
Of Caesar's death.

FIRST PLEBEIAN
I will hear Brutus speak.

SECOND PLEBEIAN
I will hear Cassius, and compare their reasons
when severally we hear them rendered.
Exit Cassius, with some of the Plebeians.

THIRD PLEBEIAN
The noble Brutus is ascended. Silence!

BRUTUS
Be patient till the last.

Romans, countrymen, and lovers, hear me for my cause, and be silent, that you may hear. Believe me for mine honour, and have respect to mine honour, that you may believe. Censure me in your wisdom, and awake your senses, that you may the better judge. If there be any in this assembly, any dear friend of Caesar's, to him

I say that Brutus' love to Caesar was no less than his. If then that friend demand why Brutus rose against Caesar, this is my answer: Not that I loved Caesar less, but that I loved Rome more. Had you rather Caesar were living, and die all slaves, than that Caesar were dead, to live all freemen? As Caesar loved me, I weep for him; as he was fortunate, I rejoice at it; as he was valiant, I honour him; but – as he was ambitious, I slew him. There is tears for his love; joy for his fortune; honour for his valour; and death for his ambition. Who is here so base that would be a bondman? If any, speak; for him have I offended. Who is here so rude that would not be a Roman? If any, speak; for him have I offended. Who is here so vile that will not love his country? If any, speak; for him have I offended. I pause for a reply.

ALL

None, Brutus, none!

BRUTUS

Then none have I offended. I have done no more to Caesar than you shall do to Brutus. The question of his death is enrolled in the Capitol; his glory not extenuated, wherein he was worthy; nor his offences enforced, for which he suffered death.

Enter Mark Antony [and others], with Caesar's body.

William Shakespeare, *Julius Caesar*, Act 3 Scenes 1 and 2

ETHICAL ANALYSIS

In earlier chapters we have been considering the question, 'In what does morality consist?' That is, on the assumption that a person wants to do what is morally right or wants to be a good person, we have gone on to ask how that aim might be achieved. Thus we looked at cultural moral relativism. This is a theory concerning the rightness or wrongness of action. Roughly, it tells us that one ought to perform a particular action if everyone in one's cultural group performs that kind of action, and that one ought not to do it if they don't. So – according to cultural relativism – I should not commit cannibalism if I am a middle-class Australian living in the early 21st century, but I should eat other people if I am a New Guinean highlander living in the 19th century. Similarly, the utilitarian and deontological theories, and Bernard Gert's substantivist account of morality, discussed in Chapters 1 and 3, provided guidelines for right action. A person should perform a certain action if it maximises happiness (utilitarianism) or if it is universalisable (some deontological theories) or if it accords with one or more of the basic moral principles (Gert 1998). In Chapter 4 we shifted focus from the rightness and wrongness of actions and looked at moral and immoral traits, virtues and vices. In so doing we were still fundamentally concerned with what morality consists of, albeit at the level of dispositions or habits, as opposed to morality of individual actions.

However, lurking behind the discussions in these previous chapters are at least three other types of issues. One set relates to the completeness of the description of the moral terrain. We saw that a focus on action was too narrow; character in the sense of virtues and vices also needed to be taken into account. But surely even the inclusion of virtues and vices is not sufficient. For we have said nothing of emotions, specifically moral emotions. Is not love, for example, a morally good emotion, and hate a morally bad one? The second range of issues concerns the motivation for performing a moral or immoral act; and the moral emotions, such as love and hate, clearly have motivational force. It also concerns the motivation for wanting to be a morally worthy (or unworthy) person; which is to say with having a certain set of virtuous or vicious dispositions, and indeed with having a particular emotional make-up (for example, being a compassionate person). A third range of issues is to do with moral reasoning. This is evidently connected to the first and second set of issues in that to be motivated to perform some action (for example, to desire to do it), is a *reason* for doing it. And of course desires (for example, the desire to help the needy), are one of the central features of the moral terrain.

The complexity of emotion

On a naïve view, emotions are simply pleasurable or painful *feelings* (that is, purely affective states). Thus love is a pleasurable feeling and jealousy a painful feeling. Accordingly, in the moral universe there are right and wrong actions, good and bad dispositions (virtues and vices) and there are moral and immoral emotions (understood as pleasurable and painful feelings). The emotion of love is morally good and that of hate morally bad.

Moreover, emotions can motivate both dispositions and actions. So a good or moral emotion is a feeling that is either good or bad in itself or else good or bad in virtue of the fact that it motivates right or wrong actions and/or virtuous or vicious dispositions.

This kind of naïve conception can apparently make sense of case study 5.5. Brutus was torn between two kinds of emotion, his love for Caesar and his love for Rome. The latter love was greater, and hence he was able to kill Caesar. Brutus had competing 'feelings' and one was stronger than the other.

Unfortunately this view gets itself into trouble with emotions such as love. For while love, compassion, sympathy, and indeed hate, jealousy, envy and so on, undoubtedly motivate actions and produce dispositions, they are far more complex than the naïve view can admit.

First – if we stay with Brutus' love for Rome and for Caesar – Brutus' love involves all sorts of so-called cognitive states such as beliefs, and indeed knowledge, about Rome and Caesar. One cannot love someone without *knowing* things about them. Love is not just a feeling like the pleasurable taste sensations produced by eating a bar of chocolate. Love involves cognitive states, including beliefs and also judgments. Love of someone can begin to wane once they are judged to be, say, weak, stupid, and so on.

Second, love and other emotions typically involve conative states: that is, states which motivate us towards action. These include desires and intentions. Love, for example, generally involves the desire to be with the person one loves and the intention to prevent harm to them. However, desires as such – much less intentions – are not necessarily to be identified with emotions. If, for example, a person desires to take a taxi in order to meet his lover, the person does not necessarily love, hate or otherwise have any emotion directed at the taxi or the taxi journey. Rather the taxi is simply desired as a means to an end, and therefore without any particular emotion. (It might seem that some emotions do not involve desires. For example, a general feeling of unfocussed depression might not involve any particular desire, but have the effect only of reducing the number and intensity of one's desires. But depression is a mood rather than an emotion; a mood is not necessarily directed towards any particular object, whereas an emotion must be. If we love, for example, there must be some person or object that we love, and if we are afraid, we must be afraid of something in particular.)

Third, emotions often involve an imaginative dimension. For example, Brutus' love of Rome would involve imaginative deliberations concerning its past, future, and so on. Typically images and conceptions of Rome are brought to mind and reflected on in his imagination, and all this is part and parcel of his deep emotional ties to the city. Once again we see that love is not a simple feeling that is mechanically brought before one's mind and causes particular actions.

Fourth, emotions such as love and hatred are dynamic, interpersonal states, and the subject of the emotion (that is, the person who loves or hates) thinks and reasons about – reflects on – the object of the emotion (that is, the person who is loved or hated). One person's hatred of another, for example, typically undergoes change over time and structures the subject's attitudes to, and actions in respect of, the person who is the object of the hatred. Hatred can grow or diminish and shift its points of emphasis in the context of real and imagined responses on the part of the object of that hatred.

Finally, moral emotions have a behavioural dimension; they are not simply inner mental states. Consider hatred. The behavioural dimension of hatred might only consist in facial expressions and tensed muscles; but equally it might consist in verbal abuse or even a physical attack. Here the line between what constitutes hatred and what is an expression of hatred becomes blurred. Someone possessed by hatred must be disposed to give expression to their hatred. That is, they will act on their hatred in suitable circumstances (such as when they can do so without facing overwhelming punishment or social disapproval), even if they succeed in suppressing the expression of their hatred in the circumstances they face.

The above points regarding love and hatred also hold for other moral emotions such sympathy and shame. Thus shame, for example, has cognitive, conative and affective elements. That is, it is complex, persisting, dynamic, and it involves reflection and is constituted in part by its behavioural expressions. (See case study 5.3.)

Emotion and motivation

Let us now turn to emotions as motivational states. Consider case study 5.1 concerning the Good Samaritan. The Good Samaritan helps a needy stranger from another community when the stranger's own brethren have passed him by. Here we need to distinguish between different kinds of motivation. Quite often we help our needy friends, members of our family and members of our community and nation. One reason for doing so is that it will pay to do so. A favour done today will be returned tomorrow. Someone who acts on such a reason is motivated by self-interest. Another reason, or at least motivation, is loyalty or community sentiment or even love of a friend. Feelings of love motivate us to help our friends. Again, we feel ourselves to be part of a social group and thus try to help fellow members of the group out of loyalty. However none of these motivations is relevant to the Good Samaritan. The point of the story of the Good Samaritan is that he helps a fellow human being notwithstanding the fact that the man he helps is neither a friend nor a member of his community. Indeed the Good Samaritan is a member of a community despised by the man in need. In helping the stranger the Good Samaritan evidently cannot be motivated either by self-interest or by loyalty: he is motivated purely by a compassionate concern for a fellow human being in need.

The Good Samaritan might be motivated by a sense that it was his duty to help; doing duty for the sake of duty, as deontologists such as Immanuel Kant so strongly recommend that we do. If so, we still need to distinguish the Samaritan's judgment that it was his duty to help the man, and his motivation for helping him. After all the priest presumably also knew that it was his duty to help, but nevertheless walked by without helping, apparently without sufficient motivation to do his duty. It is one thing to know one's duty, it is another to be sufficiently motivated to discharge one's duty. However the Good Samaritan may have been moved or motivated by compassion, and not by a sense of duty. The Good Samaritan might not even have asked himself, 'Is it my duty to help this man?' He may simply have felt compelled to act by his feelings of compassion. And in fact, of course, this is how the story is usually interpreted.

At any rate, we have identified a number of motivations for action, and all of them seem to involve emotions of one sort or another. These motivating emotions include feelings of loyalty, love, compassion, doing one's duty out of respect for one's duty, and so on. And all of these emotions are moral at least in the sense that they motivate action we would regard as being morally right. In some cases – such as feelings of loyalty – they are associated with habits or dispositions we regard as virtues. So perhaps the moral emotions constitute the motivations both for doing what is right and for developing the virtues.

While it may well be that the moral emotions constitute motivations for doing what is right and for developing the virtues, they are not the only kind of motivations. For conative states such as desires and intentions also motivate. The desire to be approved of, for example, can motivate a person to do his or her duty; and so can the intention to succeed in one's career.

What of cognitive states, such as moral beliefs, for example, the belief that one ought to do one's duty? Can they motivate us to act morally?

Consider the Kitty Genovese scenario in case study 5.2. Did the bystanders refrain from assisting Kitty because they did not have an appropriate moral emotion, such as compassion, or because they did not possess a sufficient relevant conative mental attitude, such as a desire to assist her? Empirical investigations of this kind of phenomenon suggests otherwise. Typically the bystanders in such cases, far from being emotionally inert are a bundle of conflicting emotions, and often ultimately become guilt-ridden. The problem is not a lack of emotional drive or a weak desire to assist, but a cognitive conflict in respect of moral responsibility. It appears that the bystanders would be far more likely to assist if they were in the situation of the Good Samaritan. That is, in the absence of an awareness of anyone else being able to assist, a person is far more likely to help, since it is clear to the person that he or she alone is morally responsible for action or inaction. The problem with Kitty Genovese-type cases seems to be that since many individuals could assist, no one person has a clear moral responsibility to do so and so, by a process of collective inaction, no one does anything. Hence the problem appears to lie not in the absence of a morally appropriate motivating emotion or desire, but rather in the absence of clear lines of moral responsibility; the problem is not an affective deficit, but cognitive confusion.

So *knowledge* by an individual that it is his or her responsibility to undertake an action can be just as important in determining whether particular actions take place, as the existence of powerful emotions or strong desires. Evidently moral action will not simply follow where people possess moral feelings and desires to do good. It also requires that they possess the right kinds of cognitive moral states such as knowledge or judgments of who is responsible for what, and what is right or wrong.

Here we can distinguish between a motivating state and a state that gives direction to that motivation. It might be suggested that the knowledge of who is responsible for assisting Kitty is not a motivating state, but merely a state, for example, the belief that the police ought to assist Kitty (say) that directs the pre-existing motivating state, for example, the desire that Kitty be assisted. On the other hand, it might be argued that affective and conative states, such as the desire that Kitty be assisted, are themselves logically dependent (at times) on cognitive states, such as the belief that strangers ought to be assisted when attacked. Moreover, on one version of this view, some cognitive states, notably moral beliefs, have motivational force in themselves.

It seems, then, that the range of motivating states can be quite diverse. Clearly, emotions, such as love and hate, motivate. However, desires also motivate, as do feelings of pleasure and pain (that are often, if not always, in part constitutive of emotions), desires and intentions. And perhaps cognitive states, such as moral beliefs, can also motivate.

The range of motivating states is diverse in another sense: some motivating states are morally good and others morally bad. Consider case study 5.4. Augustine explains how he stole fruit simply for the pleasure of doing what was wrong. This suggests that there is a feeling or pleasure associated with doing what is morally wrong, as well as one associated with doing one's duty. If these feelings or emotions are also motivations for action – and Augustine appears to suggest that the pleasure of doing what is wrong motivated his action – then we seem to have a problem. For at least some persons in some circumstances have an inherent reason to do what is morally wrong and no inherent and countervailing reason to do what is morally right.

Here we need to distinguish between there being a reason in the abstract and the person in question feeling the force of some reason. Naturally, we can point out to Augustine that he has a reason not to steal the fruit, that is, that to do so is morally wrong. Moreover, we can point out the harmful effects of his wrongdoing on others; this is a further reason not to steal the fruit. However, in the situation in question these are all reasons in the abstract. They will not influence someone who desires to do what is wrong and takes pleasure in wrong-doing, and has no concern about the effects of his actions on others; they won't be reasons for him. Such a person is not moved by moral emotions, moral desires or moral beliefs.

However, this is not all that can be said about case study 5.4. For one thing Augustine's desire to do what is wrong is not quite as abstract and general as might be thought. It is not simply a desire to do wrong, whatever wrong is. Rather it seems to be a desire to do what is forbidden; to do, that is, what some external power or authority (in this case God) has forbidden. In the light of this perhaps his doing what is forbidden is to some extent an expression of his autonomy in relation to authority. The pleasure he gets from his action derives at least in part from its involving him defying authority and celebrating his autonomy. Viewed from this perspective the action is not purely bad. This way of treating the case study brings out its moral ambiguity, including the moral ambiguity of emotions and feelings involved. Emotions and feelings are not necessarily either wholly good or wholly bad in themselves. Perhaps the same feelings of pleasure can be at one and the same time an expression of autonomy (and to that extent good) and a wilful defiance of legitimate authority (and to that extent bad).

Moreover, as Augustine demonstrates in this case study, we are able to deliberate and make judgments about our own motivations, including our emotions and desires. The naïve view makes it sound as though motivating emotions, desires and feelings are simply given, and are not susceptible of intellectual (including moral) scrutiny and judgment. But once we allow that they are so susceptible then, presumably, they are open to change. We are positioned to examine and influence our own motivating emotions, desires and beliefs, including our moral and immoral emotions. Such an overarching capacity for deliberation and judgment is sometimes referred to as our conscience. Engaging in such self-reflective deliberation may lead us, for example, to experience a painful emotion such as shame on contemplating the pleasure we took in another's downfall. This makes it less likely that we feel such pleasure when we confront the same or a similar situation again. If this is correct, then conscience is not simply another motivating feeling standing alongside other feelings such as pleasure and pain. Rather it is a kind of meta-judgmental capacity about oneself, including one's emotional makeup. As such, it is presumably primarily a *cognitive* capacity; if so, then once again motivation turns out to be (in part) a matter of cognition, and not simply emotion or desire. For conscience is much more like the thing that controls the steering wheel of the car, than it is the pistons that actually drive the crankshaft that turns the wheels and makes the car go.

Varieties of moral emotion

So, we are not just the passive subjects of emotions in the sense of feelings, which determine how we act. The emotions we feel are to some extent under our control – since they often depend on judgments that we make – and we have (or should have) the capacity to decide how we will act in response to the emotions that we do experience. This is well illustrated in case study 5.3. Jean-Jacques Rousseau certainly displays the capacity to do wrong. He lies about the theft of the ribbon, apparently motivated by a strongly-felt desire to avoid the disapproval of others. However, he also feels enormous sympathy for the girl he has thereby wronged.

Before turning to the motivation of avoiding the disapproval of others, let us consider the notion of sympathy.

There seem to be at least two kinds of sympathy. One can be sympathetic in the sense that one puts oneself in the shoes of another. Being able to do this, one views the world from the other person's perspective, and one feels to some extent what the other person feels. This psychological capacity is sometimes called empathy. Invaluable as it is, it is not a moral emotion like, say, compassion. Compassion involves wanting to do good for that person. It is not simply a matter of putting oneself in their shoes or feeling what they feel. After all, the most vicious of persons might be able to be sympathetic to someone in this sense before going on to do the person great harm.

Sympathy in the second sense involves not only feeling what someone else feels, but wanting to do them good. Rousseau has, we suggest, sympathy in both senses for the girl. Unfortunately, his sympathy, including his desire to do her good (or at least avoid harming her) is overridden by his desire to avoid the disapproval of others. Thus he ends up harming her.

However the fact that he harms her is a source of shame. Rousseau feels shame because he did what he knew he should not have done. In particular, he did what he and others know he should not have done. He feels shame because he knows that they will think him a wrongdoer if they discover what he did, and he knows that they would be right to so think of him. It is important to stress here that shame results not only from one's desire to be approved of by others, but also from one's belief that one does not deserve to be approved of by others. Because one knows one has done wrong, one knows one does not deserve to be approved of.

Let us more directly consider the desire to be approved of by others. Here we are assuming that this desire has an emotional character, including attendant feelings of pain and pleasure, so it is not, so to speak, just a mere desire. We are also assuming that this desire has an ethical dimension; we desire to be thought to be a person who is good or worthy of respect. This is not to deny that there is a simpler and closely related desire that people have to be liked by others. Nor is it to say that people do not sometimes desire respect for the wrong reasons, for example, the mafia hit-man who desires to be respected for his cold-blooded ruthlessness.

The desire to be approved of is not simply a desire and feeling with respect to one's own actions, as in the case where one eats an ice cream motivated by the pleasure to be derived from consuming it. Nor is it apparently an emotion of the sort we have discussed above, such as the feelings of concern for the safety of one's friend. For these emotions evidently involve a direct and straightforward connection between one person experiencing the emotion and another person who is the object of the emotional attitude. Rather Rousseau's desire to avoid disapproval is, in the first place, an attitude with respect to the attitudes of others, and in the second place, an attitude with respect to their attitude to him. It is a kind of second order attitude: an attitude about an attitude. But it is also an attitude (albeit a second order one), which has as its ultimate object oneself. If such second order attitudes (about oneself) can motivate actions, then they may do so in a more complex and roundabout way than ordinary first order attitudes or emotions, such as the desire to help others.

At any rate these kinds of motivating emotions – if that is what they are – raise questions about our motivations not only for acting in a certain way, but for trying to be a certain kind of person rather than some other kind of person. For example, these sorts of second order motivations raise questions about our reasons for trying to have virtues such as courage or honesty or whatever. It should be noted that these kinds of second order attitudes can conflict with one another. It is one thing to desire to be approved of by others, it is another (as Kant points out) to want to be good; and still another to actually be good. On occasion, one can only be good by doing what the social group to which one belongs disapproves of.

Moral reasoning

The various approaches to morality we have examined all claim to help us in our reasoning about morality. In fact, they claim to help us in both of the major forms of reasoning: so-called *theoretical reasoning*, and *practical reasoning*. Theoretical reasoning is reasoning about what is the case, about what is true. The aim of theoretical reasoning is to produce true beliefs. Practical reasoning is reasoning about what we ought to *do*. The aim of practical reasoning is to guide us to rational action. We typically act in order to achieve outcomes that we take to be valuable. A practically rational action, then, will be one that produces the greatest, or at least sufficient, value. There is, of course, a variety of different values, including moral value as well as prudential value, financial value, aesthetic value and so on. (We discuss the relationship between different values below.)

Though theoretical and practical reasoning are importantly different from each other, they are also intimately connected. In particular, when we are trying to decide what to do we usually have to draw on the results of theoretical reasoning. We must discover what courses of action are available to us, and we must work out what the likely consequences of those various actions are, and these are both matters of fact. In other words, we are only likely to be able to act rationally if we have true beliefs.

Both theoretical and practical reasoning can be seen as involving a two-step process (Alexandra, Matthews and Miller 2002). Firstly, we should work out the considerations relevant to the issue at hand. Then we should decide what to believe (in the case of theoretical reasoning) or what to do (in the case of practical reasoning) on the basis of these considerations. The form of such a process is made explicit in the production of 'arguments'. Here the term 'argument' refers not to a heated disagreement, but rather to a certain kind of structure of sentences. In philosophical terminology, the considerations supposedly relevant to the matter are put in sentences called 'premises', while the sentences that represent the decisions we make on the basis of those considerations are referred to as 'conclusions'.

Consider the following example of an argument, which Rousseau might have put forth in the situation described in case study 5.3.

- Premise 1: I have stolen a ribbon and it is found on my person.
- Premise 2: I have been asked how I came to be in possession of it.
- Premise 3: Stealing and lying are both immoral.
- Premise 4: I do not want to act immorally.
- Conclusion: I tell the truth.

Reflecting the two-step process of reasoning outlined above, there is a two-step process for assessing arguments. Firstly we need to look at the premises: do we have sufficient reason to accept them, and have we included all relevant considerations? Secondly, we need to look at the relationship between the premises and the conclusions. Do the premises actually provide support for the conclusion, or as it is often put, does the conclusion follow from the premises? A good argument, then, is one that contains only premises which we have good reason to accept, and all such premises which are relevant to the issue at hand, and where the conclusion does follow from those premises.

As mentioned earlier, a variety of values exist, including moral and prudential value and, at least on the face of it, these different considerations will occasionally compete. If we try to act in such a way as to promote an outcome that is valuable in one way – say in terms of promoting our self-interest – we may make it impossible to act in a way that will bring about an outcome that is valuable in another way – fulfilling our moral obligations, for example – and vice versa. In such situations we are faced with a conflict between two types of practical reasons, deriving from two (and sometimes more than two) kinds of value or principle. Consider in this connection Rousseau's situation in case study 5.3.

Above we presented an argument that Rousseau had reasons to tell the truth about how the missing ribbon came into his possession. These were moral reasons. But it is also clear from Rousseau's account that he had other reasons – prudential or self-interested reasons – *not* to tell the truth. In the light of this conflict, Rousseau must decide which sort of reason is the more compelling. How is he to do that? Some people think that moral considerations should always take precedence over other sorts of values when there is a conflict between them. This seems implausible, however. We can certainly imagine circumstances in which the performance of a self-interested action results in the production of more value than the moral costs of failing to perform the morally right action. Consider a case where you are stopped by a stranger who, slightly distressed, asks you for directions. Knowing that there are other people who can provide these directions, and knowing also that you will miss your train to the last showing of a film you very much want to see, it seems that the prudent course of action is to ignore (politely) the needs of the stranger. In such a case more value is promoted by acting out of self-interest, rather than acting in the interests of the stranger.

Not only are there cases of practical reasoning where decision-making is difficult because the reasons derived from different values pull us in different directions, we can, it seems, find ourselves facing situations where reasons derived from the same kind of value can come into conflict. For example, commonly we find that we seem to have a moral reason to do a certain action, and also a moral reason not to do that action. Consider Brutus in case study 5.5. He is (apparently) torn between his friendship for Caesar and his loyalty to Rome. Obviously he cannot act on both reasons; he must choose between them. This kind of situation, where we have moral reasons to act in two incompatible ways, is often described as a moral dilemma.

Much of the difference between various moral theories comes down to disagreements about what kinds of considerations are in fact relevant in practical reasoning about moral matters. Utilitarians, for example, think that the only considerations that should be taken into account are those which bear on the consequences of actions; presumably in the case of Brutus, violation of loyalty would be given little or no weight relative to the likely good and bad consequences of assassinating Caesar. Some deontologists, on the other hand, would say that these consequences should not be given any weight; all that matters here is Brutus' duties.

On the kind of pluralist approach favoured in this work, a whole range of reasons can be relevant to moral decisions and should be taken into account in making such decisions. These will include duties and consequences, but may also include (reflectively endorsed) emotions, desires and the like.

Readings

Alexandra, Andrew, Matthews, Steve and Miller, Seumas (2002) *Reasons, Values and Institutions*, Tertiary Press, Melbourne.

Augustine (1963) *The Confessions of St Augustine*, Rex Warner (translator), Mentor, New York, Book 2, Ch 1.

Blum, Lawrence (1980) 'Compassion' in Rorty, Amelie Oksenberg (ed) *Explaining Emotions*, University of California Press, Berkeley.

Casey, John (1990) *Pagan Virtue: An Essay in Ethics*, Oxford University Press, Oxford, pp 9-28.

Hume, David (1978) 'Of the origin of the natural virtues and vices' in Nidditch, Peter (ed) *A Treatise of Human Nature*, Clarendon Press, Oxford, pp 514-28.

Kant, Immanuel (1989) 'Jealousy, envy and spite' in Sommers, Christina, and Sommers, Fred (eds) *Vice and Virtue in Everyday Life: Introductory Readings in Ethics*, Harcourt Brace Jovanovich, San Diego, pp 404-12.

McGuire, Martin (1963) 'On conscience', *Journal of Philosophy*, vol 60, no 10, pp 253-63.

Oakley, Justin (1992) *Morality and the Emotions*, Routledge, London.

Rousseau, Jean-Jacques (1781, 1953) *The Confessions*, Penguin, Harmondsworth, pp 86-89.

Sartre, Jean-Paul (1962) *Sketch for a Theory of the Emotions*, Mairet, P (translator), Methuen, London.

Sehleff, Leon Shaskolsky (1978) *The Bystander; Behaviour, Law, Ethics*, Lexington Books, Lexington Mass, pp 1-2.

Shakespeare, William (1988) *Julius Caesar*, Bloom, Harold (ed), Chelsea House, New York, Act 3 Scenes 1 and 2.

Strawson, Peter Frederick (1974) 'Freedom and resentment' in Strawson, Peter Frederick (ed) *Freedom and Resentment, and Other Essays*, Methuen, London.

Taylor, Gabriele (1985) *Pride, Shame and Guilt: Emotions of Self-Assessment*, Oxford University Press, Oxford.

Wilson, James (1993) 'Sympathy' in Wilson, James (ed) *The Moral Sense*, Free Press, New York, pp 29-54.

6: Professional role morality

Mrs Smith's vital signs were almost non-existent when Wayne found her slumped in the bathroom. What should he do? He knew where the keys to the drugs cupboard were kept, and he was sure that he was capable of administering the life-saving injection. Wayne paused: they had been told often enough that only the qualified medical staff were allowed to administer injections. If an orderly like Wayne was found doing so it was instant dismissal. But surely the rationale for the prohibition was to make it more likely that people would get the best possible treatment – if Wayne didn't take matters into his own hands Mrs Smith might well be dead by the time the medical staff got there.

Provided by the authors

CASE STUDY 6.2

Consider the case of a doctor who falls among thieves, or better still, terrorists. They have forty hostages whom the leader, con-

94

veniently suffering from acute appendicitis, has decided to kill. The doctor will be spared on account of his usefulness. There is some dissension in the camp however and the second in command would prefer to release them as a public relations gesture. If the leader dies there's a very good chance the second in command will take over and release them. We'll assume that the doctor has the trust of the group and could convince them that the death was an accident and so save himself from any possible recriminations. The hostages are innocent, not politicians, soldiers, nor anyone the terrorists could argue are directly opposed to them or contributing, even negatively, to their plight, whatever it is.

John Harris (1980) *Violence and Responsibility*

John Harris (1980) *Violence and Responsibility*

CASE STUDY 6.3

Let us consider this waiter in the cafe. His movement is quick and forward, a little too precise, a little too rapid. He comes towards the patrons with a step a little too quick. He bends forward a little too eagerly; his voice, his eyes, express an interest a little too solicitous for the order of the customer. Finally there he returns, trying to imitate in his walk the inflexible stiffness of some kind of automaton while carrying his tray with the recklessness of tight-rope walker by putting it in a perpetually unstable, perpetually broken equilibrium which he perpetually re-establishes by a light movement of the arm and hand. All his behaviour seems to us a game. He applies himself to chaining his movements as if they were mechanisms, the one regulating the other; his gestures and even his voice seem to be mechanisms; he gives himself the quickness and pitiless rapidity of things. He is playing, he is amusing himself. But what is he playing? We need not watch long before we can explain it: he is playing at being a waiter in a cafe. There is nothing there to surprise us. The game is a kind of marking out and investigation. The child plays with his body in order to explore it, to take inventory of it; the waiter in the cafe plays with his condition in order to realise it. This obligation is not different from that which is imposed on all tradesmen. Their condition is wholly one of ceremony. The public demands of them that they realise it as a ceremony; there is the dance of the grocer, of the tailor, of the auctioneer, by which they endeavour to persuade their clientele that they are nothing but a grocer, an auctioneer, a tailor. A grocer who dreams is offensive to the buyer, because such a grocer is not wholly a grocer. Society demands that he limits himself to his function as a grocer, just as the soldier at attention makes himself into a soldier-thing with a direct regard which does not see at all, which is no longer meant to see, since it is the rule and not the interest of the moment which determines the point he must fix his eyes on (the sight 'fixed at ten paces'.) There are indeed many precautions to imprison a man in what he is, as if we lived in perpetual fear that he might escape from it, that he might break away and elude his condition.

Jean-Paul Sartre (1956) *Being and Nothingness*

CASE STUDY 6.4

The most reflective of the accounts I have found is by an Italian soldier who fought the Austrians in World War I: Emilio Lussu, later a socialist leader and anti-fascist exile. Lussu, then a lieutenant, together with a corporal, had moved during the night into a position overlooking the Austrian trenches. He watched the Austrians having morning coffee and felt a kind of amazement, as if he had not expected to find anything human in the enemy lines.

> Those strongly defended trenches, which we had attacked
> so many times without success had ended by seeming to us
> inanimate, like desolate buildings uninhabited by men, the
> refuge only of mysterious and terrible beings of whom we knew
> nothing. Now they were showing themselves to us as they really
> were, men and soldiers like us, in uniform like us, moving about,
> talking and drinking coffee, just as our own companions behind
> us were doing at that moment.

A young officer appears and Lussu takes aim at him; then the Austrian lights a cigarette and Lussu pauses. 'This cigarette formed an invisible link between us. No sooner did I see its smoke than I wanted a cigarette myself …' Behind perfect cover, he has time to think about his decision. He felt the war justified, 'a hard necessity'. He recognised that he had obligations to the men under his command. 'I knew it was my duty to fire.' And yet he did not. He hesitated, he writes, because the Austrian officer was so entirely oblivious to the danger that threatened him.

> I reasoned like this: To lead a hundred, even a thousand, men against another hundred, or thousand was one thing; but to detach one man from the rest and say to him, as it were: 'Don't move, I'm going to shoot you. I'm going to kill' – that was different … To fight is one thing, but to kill a man is another. And to kill him like that is to murder him.

Lussu turned to his corporal … 'Look here – I'm not going to fire on a man alone like that. Will you?' … 'No, I won't either.' Here the line has been clearly drawn between the member of an army who makes war together with his comrades and the individual who stands alone. Lussu objected to stalking a human prey. What else, however, does a sniper do?

Michael Walzer (1984) *Just and Unjust Wars*

CASE STUDY 6.5

Nora Tomorrow I'm going home – to what used to be my home, I mean. It will be easier for me to find something to do there.

Helmer Oh, you blind, inexperienced …

Nora I must set about getting experience, Torvald.

Helmer And leave your home, your husband and your children? Don't you care what people will say?

Nora That's no concern of mine. All I know is that this is necessary for me.

Helmer This is outrageous! You are betraying your most sacred duty.

Nora And what do you consider to be my most sacred duty?

Helmer Does it take me to tell you that? Isn't it your duty to your husband and your children?

Nora I have another duty equally sacred.

Helmer You have not. What duty might that be?

Nora My duty to myself.

Helmer First and foremost, you are a wife and mother.

Nora That I don't believe any more. I believe that first and foremost I am an individual, just as much as you are – or at least I'm going to try to be. I know most people agree with you, Torvald, and that's also what it says in books. I have to think things out for myself, and get things clear.

Helmer You are talking like a child. You understand nothing about the society you live in.

Nora No, I don't. But I shall go into that too. I must try to discover who is right, society or me.

Henrik Ibsen (1961) *A Doll's House*

ETHICAL ANALYSIS

Each of us is at the same time a unique individual, and the occupant of a number of social roles. These roles can be of first importance to us, helping to shape our self-understanding. Consider the waiter described by Jean-Paul Sartre in case study 6.3. He is not simply carrying out a series of tasks, his behaviour is that of someone who has taken on a role and is acting it out. Moreover, the taking on of a social role is not simply a matter of external behaviour. The social role player has internalised a set of attitudes associated with his or her role. For Sartre's waiter, being a waiter has become a defining aspect of his persona.

Occupational roles are not the only kinds of social roles. As shown in case study 6.5, being a mother or father is also to some extent a social role, as is being a friend, a neighbour, a citizen and so on. We can see also that there are various social expectations that certain people will occupy certain roles; women will come to play the role of mothers and wives, for example. However case study 6.5 also illustrates the point that we can choose to reject particular social roles society seeks to impose on us. Evidently we are not simply automatons being pushed by the forces of social role formation; now this way, and now that.

Social roles are in part defined by social norms. Social norms are (roughly) principles governing behaviour that happen to be followed by the members of some social group, and that are regarded as having moral weight. Thus telling the truth is a social norm in our society. We believe we are under a moral obligation to tell the truth, and by and large people do tell the truth. Again there is a social norm in our society not to kill people. We believe we ought not kill other human beings, except in exceptional circumstances such as self-defence.

Naturally, we need to distinguish between the existence of a social norm and the existence of an objective moral obligation. It is always open to us to question whether or not a social norm is, as a matter of objective fact, morally right. For example, in case study 6.5 Nora disputes the validity of social norms in her society. And as we saw in Chapter 2, there are grounds for thinking that social norms ought not be identified with what is morally right. Society can get things horribly morally wrong.

So social roles are defined in part by particular social norms. But there are different social roles, and therefore varying social norms and expectations associated with these roles. The role of a doctor is different from that of a waiter, and the moral obligations of doctors are not the same as those of waiters. Doctors are under an obligation to provide people with medical assistance, whereas waiters are under an obligation to provide table service. A doctor who insisted on bringing her patient cups of tea and sandwiches, but avoided medical examinations or medical advice would be morally culpable. Similarly, a waiter who refused to bring the menu or the food one had ordered, but rather insisted on providing medical advice and on writing prescriptions on the bill for the meal, would be taken to have abrogated his duty. (Indeed he might even be taken to be insane.)

The existence of social roles with distinctive duties raises a question. What is the relationship between, on the one hand, the moral rights and obligations of social roles – especially clearly defined occupational and professional roles – and on the other the moral rights and obligations of so-called ordinary morality? Here 'ordinary morality' designates the morality that governs our actions when we are not functioning in accordance with some occupational or professional role; or indeed perhaps not in accordance with any given social role.

There are two main schools of thought about the relation between so-called ordinary morality and role morality. Some believe that role morality is a distinctive kind of morality, with its own justification and demands. On this view, at least some of the time the demands of role morality and ordinary morality can come into conflict. According to other theorists, there is no distinction between ordinary morality and role morality.

Those who deny the distinction between ordinary morality and role morality acknowledge that certain actions are usually required of people in certain roles and not of those who do not have those roles. They claim, however, that this does not show that the moral demands made of role-occupants differ in kind from those made on others. No doubt a waiter should not generally offer medical advice or engage in medical treatment of the sick, and a doctor should. This, however, is not because of some special morality that applies only to doctors, say. It is rather because the doctor possesses a special competence that the waiter lacks. Everyone has an obligation to help those in extreme need if they can. This applies to waiters just as much as to doctors. However, because the doctor is so much better equipped to help than the waiter, and because the waiter may do more harm than good, the waiter should generally make way for the doctor. Sometimes, however, there is no doctor available, and other people may be able to help. This is the kind of situation described in case study 6.1. Since Mrs Smith will probably die if Wayne does not provide her with medical help, and will probably live if he does, then he is obliged to give her that help. If he does not, he cannot justify himself by claiming that it was not his role to do so, according to those who deny the distinction between role and ordinary morality.

Similarly, doctors usually should use their medical expertise to help people become well, rather than using it to kill them. But again this is not because of some special role morality that applies only to doctors. No-one should kill others unless there are very good reasons to do so. If there are such reasons then people may be *required* to kill; doctors as much as others. In case study 6.2 the doctor has the chance to kill a terrorist, thereby saving the lives of 40 innocent people. He cannot justify his failure to kill the terrorist by appealing to the alleged prohibition on harming his patients.

In recent discussions, probably the more popular position has been that there are distinctive role moralities, and that the demands of these moralities can come into conflict with the demands of ordinary morality. Consider case study 6.4, where the sniper is faced with the apparent role obligation as a soldier to shoot his enemy. Yet ordinary morality appears to dictate that he not shoot the soldier on the other side of enemy lines. The soldier is rather, from the perspective of ordinary morality, another human being out on an innocent morning stroll. As such he has a right to life, which other people are obliged to respect. The sniper, it is true, tried to rationalise his failure to kill the enemy soldier by in effect claiming that stalking a human prey is not part of the soldier's role. Yet as Michael Walzer tellingly asks 'What else does a sniper do?' In fact, what seems to be going on here is that because of the ordinariness of the activities engaged in by the sniper's target, he finds himself unable to fully engage himself in his role and its demands, but rather is reminded of the requirements of ordinary morality as it applies simply between human beings. Though we may sympathise with the soldier here, say those who support the idea of a distinctive role morality, the simple truth is that if he fails to take the opportunity presented to him to shoot a member of the enemy army he is, as a soldier, failing to do what he should do.

As we will see in later chapters, there can be conflicts between the demands of role morality and those of ordinary morality in relation to professional requirements such as confidentiality. For example, the social worker, Margaret 'Peggy' Langhammer (case study 8.4) went to jail rather than breach confidentiality. She claimed that she has a moral obligation of confidentiality to a rape victim in virtue of the rape victim being her client. However, the accused rapist wanted access to her files so he could prepare his defence. Apparently, other people – say, police officers who may have interviewed the rape victim – would not necessarily have this special obligation of confidentiality. There is no general presumption of confidentiality in discussions that people have with each other, and in this case there are strong moral reasons why the contents of the discussion should be made available. Without them the court will not have access to important information relevant to their deliberations regarding a serious crime, and their lack could lead to a grave injustice being done to the accused. Langhammer's refusal to offer up the information she has depends in effect on claiming that questions such as the possibility of such injustice should have no bearing on her deliberations in her role as a social worker. The only factor she should consider is the welfare of her clients, actual and potential: the effects of her actions on others who are not her clients simply do not enter the picture.

There appear to be strong grounds for accepting the distinction between ordinary and role morality. In any case, we will accept this distinction here. It follows that sometimes the demands of ordinary morality, on the one hand, and role morality, on the other, can come into conflict with each other. And, as we have argued is the case with other such moral conflicts, one of these demands does not automatically take precedence over the other. It seems more plausible to think that sometimes one should win out and sometimes the other, depending on the circumstances. For example, Wayne in case study 6.1 should disregard the regulations governing his occupation and assist the woman. But equally, in other cases, one's professional obligations may override the dictates of ordinary morality, as in the case of the sniper.

So far we have worked with a relatively untheorised notion of role morality. Here we wish to explore more deeply this notion. To simplify matters we will speak only of one species of role morality, namely professional morality.

The ethical dimension of any given professional practice has what might be called an internal and an external aspect. Two things need to be noted about the external ethical aspect. Firstly, it consists of moral principles that ought to be adhered to by the occupant of the professional role. But secondly, these moral principles are typically not necessary – and certainly not sufficient – for the professional to undertake that practice competently.

These external moral principles – and their associated character traits (virtues) – have such a high degree of generality that they exist more or less independently of any particular professional practice. Such principles and virtues govern behaviour and attitudes in most professional behaviour, indeed in most areas of human activity. For example, the principles not to steal or take innocent human life, or the virtues of honesty and diligence, apply in all areas of life. Many such moral principles are enshrined in the law. Thus it is against the law to commit murder, to steal or to engage in fraud. When people engage in such activities in their professional capacity, the breach of law and morality is likely to be seen as particularly serious.

The internal ethical aspect consists of principles and virtues which are necessary for a professional to undertake his or her particular professional practice competently. These may vary widely from profession to profession. Thus, manual dexterity is a virtue which is internal to the profession of surgery, but by no means to most professions; suspicion is a virtue in a detective, but not in a minister of religion, and so on.

No sharp line divides the internal from the external ethical aspects in any particular profession. The distinction is nevertheless an important one for us to make here, for discussions concerning professional ethics are sometimes conducted as if the ethical dimension to professional life consisted wholly of its external aspect. Of course – it is sometimes argued – professionals as well as, say, neighbours ought not to endanger life or commit fraud, but no separate set of moral considerations applies to professionals but not to neighbours. Naturally – the argument continues – there are standards of professional practice that are particular to a given profession; but professional practice is one thing and morality another. The existence of the internal ethical aspect undermines this argument. Morality is internal to professional practice.

This is not to say that all aspects of professional practice are matters of morality. That would be absurd. It might be unprofessional for lawyers to wear shabby clothing when appearing in court or for doctors to be unsympathetic to their patients, but it is not necessarily immoral. On the other hand, some practices that are internal to a given profession are matters of morality, and not because they violate some externally determined moral principle. For example, if a policeman fails to intervene in an attempted burglary, the policeman has not only failed in his professional duty, he is also morally culpable. Similarly, a doctor is morally culpable if he or she fails to attend to a patient who is very ill. Moreover, they are morally culpable if they fail to keep abreast of relevant developments in medical science. Not doing so demonstrates not simply technical incompetence, but moral failure.

In undertaking a particular profession, then, individuals accept professional obligations, but some of these professional obligations are also moral obligations. These moral obligations are additional to the moral obligations that they had prior to entering the profession; they are internal to the profession.

A number of questions concerning the internal ethical aspect of the professions now arise. One of these issues concerns moral basis of professional roles. A second issue concerns the moral obligations incumbent on someone in that role.

Moral basis of professional roles and the duty to aid

That professionals have a range of special duties (and rights) seems undeniable. Such duties are recognised in popular attitudes, professional codes of ethics, and the law. The question we address here is: 'Where do these duties come from?'

One approach is to see them as arising in just the same way as many other special duties do; generated by the actions of the individuals who have them. We can act in a number of ways to generate such duties. Here we consider two that have been appealed to as the basis of professional duties: making promises and creating reasonable expectations.

We commonly create special duties through promising. There is no general duty to give money to the charity World Vision, for example, but if I have signed a document promising that I will give $50 each month to that charity, then I have a duty to do so. Similarly, some have claimed, professionals come to have a range of special duties by (in effect) promising to act in certain ways on entering the profession. At least some of these promises will be explicitly made through a 'swearing in' process. Often, they are tacit: it is understood that they 'come with the territory'. However, even if this is an adequate description of what actually happens, it does not provide an adequate account of the basis of professional duties. For do professionals have any obligation to make such promises?

Consider the following kind of case. Social workers have a duty to keep information they obtain from their clients confidential. This duty is much stronger than the requirements of ordinary morality. A particular social worker might explain his being under such an obligation by referring to his acceptance of a code of ethics or the like. But what if someone sets themselves up as a social worker and announces that they have no intention of being bound by the kind of stringent requirements of confidentiality that most of his colleagues accept? He points out that he has made no promise to accept those requirements, so has no duty to do so, since such duties are consequent on promises. If the response is, as it is likely to be, that he is required to make such a promise, then it is not really the promise that is the basis of the duty, but the duty that is the reason for the promise. Promises might be useful in making explicit what is required of professionals and bringing home to them the importance of their duties, but they do not appear to be the ultimate basis for those duties.

Promising is not the only way in which we can act to create special duties, however. Sometimes we do so by acting in ways which generate reasonable expectations by others. (Promising is, in fact, one, but not the only way, of doing this.) If, for example, I have cooked a meal for my aged, bed-ridden neighbour every night for the last five years, then she has a reasonable expectation that I will do so tonight, unless I inform her otherwise. Arguably, in this sort of case, I have come to have a duty to provide her with her evening meal; it is not just that I am acting well in doing so, but that I would be acting badly if I failed to do so (unless I made alternative arrangements etc).

It has been suggested that professional duties are to be explained in the same way. Once a person actually takes on a role to (say) assist those who are ill, reasonable expectations are generated on the part of the ill that their illnesses will be treated. As a consequence a doctor comes to have a duty to treat those who are ill. This suggestion is akin to the view that professional duties are based on promises: in both cases the duties are generated by an action that is not itself obligatory. However, again, the notion of creating expectations that one will assist does not seem sufficient to generate a moral obligation to assist, unless there is some prior moral obligation to assist. Consider a winemaker. The winemaker has no moral obligation to make and sell wine to a community, but in fact the winemaker does make and sell wine to the community. Accordingly, the members of the community reasonably assume that they will continue to procure wine from the winemaker, albeit at a price. Now assume that the winemaker decides that while he will continue to make wine, he will do so in smaller quantities and only for selected customers; those who understand and fully appreciate wine, as distinct from ordinary drinkers. Accordingly, the reasonable expectations of many former customers – the non-connoisseurs – are dashed. Moreover, since there is no other winemaker to whom they have access, these customers suffer various harms, notably deprivation of pleasure. Notwithstanding this deprivation, surely the winemaker does not have a *moral duty* to make and sell wine to ordinary drinkers. Certainly, given his limited stocks of wine, he is discriminating against the ordinary drinkers in favour of the connoisseurs, but this discrimination is not arbitrary; indeed it has a certain rational justifiability. We conclude that the mere creation by a role occupant of reasonable expectations that he will provide benefits does not generate a moral duty to so provide those benefits.

In our view, attempts to base the content of professional duties on the actions of individual professionals are inadequate. Even if some such account might be adequate as an explanation as to why some individual role occupant, such as a fireman, has a duty to (say) put out fires, it does not provide a moral basis for the institutional role itself. So it does not provide a moral basis for fire brigades and the associated institutional role of fireman. Specifically, it does not acknowledge that there is a moral requirement to see to it that there are fire brigades and firemen to extinguish fires in order to avert the very serious harms of uncontained fires. Indeed, it seems that it cannot do so. On such accounts, if no-one chooses to assume the role of fireman, or in some other way generate reasonable expectations that they can be relied on to put out fires, and no-one else chooses to put out fires, then no-one has done a moral wrong and, in particular, no-one has failed to act in accordance with their moral duty. We believe, on the contrary that there is a moral duty to see that fires are put out, a moral duty which was not being discharged in this case. (And of course, this point can be generalised to a range of professional roles.)

Professionals – and their duties – cannot be understood in purely individualistic terms. Professionals are members of institutions. To understand the nature of professional role morality we need to examine the moral basis for the creation of institutions and the consequent institutional moral duties to assist, incumbent on members of those institutions (Alexandra and Miller 2003, 2009; Miller 2009).

As we pointed out in Chapter 3, it is generally accepted that an individual should help others where she is the only one able to do so and there is minimal cost involved. The same holds true of groups; there are collective responsibilities. Consider the following scenario. A group of bushwalkers comes across an incipient grass fire in the bush which – given the very high temperature and strong winds – will, if not extinguished, develop into a full-scale bush fire that will destroy property, and perhaps even lead to loss of life. No single member of the group could put out the small grass fire, but if they act jointly they can do so without risk to themselves, or indeed any great inconvenience. Moreover, they know that there is no way for them to warn the local community of the impending danger, should they refrain from extinguishing the fire. It seems that, given their awareness of the near certainty of a conflagration if they do not intervene, the members of the group have a collective moral responsibility to do so.

So the need of groups for various forms of assistance that can only be adequately rendered by other groups generates collective responsibilities on the part of groups that can assist. Moreover, where such collective responsibilities can most effectively be discharged by establishing institutions and institutional roles whose institutional duties consist of providing such aid, for example, fire brigades and firemen (or doctors and hospitals, and so on), then members of the group who have the collective responsibility have a derivative responsibility to establish and support such institutions.

Further, members of a given group may have collective moral responsibilities towards the membership of that very group, that is, the group of which they are members. Assume that there is a high probability of bushfires destroying the property and taking the life of some very small percentage of Australia's population, but that with respect to any individual Australian the risk is close to zero. In this situation all or most Australians have a collective moral responsibility to prevent bushfires, and that responsibility can be discharged at minimal cost and inconvenience to any individual Australian. However, from the perspective of narrow individual self-interest, each Australian would not contribute. In the first place, given the almost zero possibility of harm to his or her self-interest, each does not have an incentive to contribute to a cooperative fire prevention scheme. And in the second place, even if such a cooperative scheme existed, self interest would dictate that each putative participant free-ride. We conclude that the fire prevention activity in question is undertaken in large part as a consequence of a perceived collective moral responsibility, and might initially take the form of local volunteer fire prevention associations. In due course, a division of labour tends to evolve, and the institution of professional fire brigades is established to discharge the collective moral responsibility to avoid the harms caused by fires.

The (collective) duty to assist may, then, in certain cases, imply the duty to establish and support institutions with specialised role holders to achieve the object of the duty (Miller 2009). Once we have discharged that duty we may generally have no further duty to assist within the area of the institutions' operations. Indeed, generally we should not even *try* to assist, given our relative lack of expertise and the likelihood that we will get in the way of the role holders. Still, on occasions when no role holder is available and we possess relevant capacities, the individual or collective duty becomes re-animated (Alexandra and Miller 2005).

To understand the specific content of professional role morality, then, we need to examine the purposes that the various professions have been formed to serve, and the way in which professional roles must be constructed in order to achieve those purposes. Of course, one only comes to have a professional role through voluntary action, but the morality that comes with that role is not itself ultimately grounded on the individual's choice.

Professional role obligations

Once institutions and their constitutive roles have been established on some adequate moral basis, such as the duty to aid, then those who undertake these roles necessarily put themselves under obligations of various kinds; obligations that attach to, and are in part constitutive of, those roles. Let us consider three dimensions of such role obligations, namely, competence, negligence, and individual versus collective responsibility.

Normally, we cannot be blamed for not doing something if we were not capable of doing it. As the saying has it 'Ought implies can.' However, those who undertake professional roles are, in effect, asserting that they are competent to carry out the tasks that are associated with those roles. Someone who has been accredited and sets themselves up as a surgeon is assumed to be competent to undertake surgery. If they do not have the skill and knowledge to carry out some operation they undertake, they are not excused from moral blame on the grounds that they were not able to perform the operation successfully. Given our reliance on professionals, and the amount of harm they can inflict if they are incompetent, it is a serious moral fault to undertake a professional role without demonstrable competence.

However, many breaches of role obligations do not involve incompetence. It is possible for, say, a competent accountant nevertheless to be negligent in the monitoring of various banking activities for which he or she is responsible. The claim here would not be that the accountant was incompetent to undertake the accountant's role, but rather that he did not exercise that competence when in that role. Similar points can be made in respect of lawyers, doctors, social workers and so on.

Once again, the moral significance of recklessness and negligence will vary from one professional context to another. It is no doubt foolish, but it is not morally wrong, for a gambler to be reckless or negligent with his or her own money. But the question that needs to be asked is whether or not ongoing recklessness and negligence is morally problematic – as opposed to being merely foolish – for a lawyer in charge of other people's money. The answer is presumably that it is. Just as an inability to competently undertake the professional role of a doctor, welfare worker, lawyer, director, banker and so on, is likely to cause enormous harm to patients, clients, depositors, shareholders, so recklessness in the provision of their relevant services, is likely to cause great harm also.

The point here is that these professional obligations are also moral obligations. They are moral obligations in virtue of the magnitude of the harm to clients that is likely to ensue if these professional obligations are not properly discharged.

A final issue here concerns ascribing responsibility within an institutional framework. As a matter of fact, much of the work professionals do occurs within large institutions such as hospitals, government departments, industrial concerns and the like. In such settings, outcomes are typically the result of numerous actions by many people. Accordingly, individuals have a tendency to fail to see themselves as responsible for the outcomes of the collective activity of the institution. This is especially prevalent in a professional context of negligence, incompetence and non-adherence to established procedures.

These responsibilities – responsibilities that, as we have seen, are moral as well as professional – do not cease to be real merely because they are ignored. In the first place, each member of a collective entity, such as a committee or board of directors, has a responsibility to follow established procedures. For example, an individual banker ought not approve large loans without the appropriate supporting documentation.

In the second place, the notion of collective responsibility entails that the decisions of the collective as a whole are the responsibility of each individual member, whether that member in fact influenced those decisions or not (Miller 2001). For example, if the driving force behind a dubious research proposal is one member of an ethics committee, this does not absolve other members for responsibility for the proposal being approved.

In the third place, no individual member of a collective such as a committee or board of directors is absolved of his or her moral responsibilities merely because those around him or her are failing to discharge theirs. If individual members are able effectively to oppose irresponsible conduct or to resign, then those people who choose not to take either of these courses of action are morally responsible for the actions of the group.

We can conclude that the ethical dimension is quite central to 'normal' professional practice. The professions are not simply activities driven by financial and other rewards to those individuals who engage in them. They are also activities which are, in part, governed by professional responsibilities which are also moral responsibilities.

Readings

Alexandra, Andrew and Miller, Seumas (2003) 'Needs, moral self-consciousness and professional roles' in Rowan, John and Zinaich, Samuel (eds) *Ethics for the Professions*, Wadsworth, Belmont, pp 134–40.

— (2005) 'Common morality and "institutionalising" ethics', *Australian Journal of Professional and Applied Ethics*, vol 7, no 1, pp 24–33.

— (2009) 'Ethical theory, "common morality" and professional obligations', *Theoretical Medicine and Bioethics*, vol 30, no 1, pp 69–80.

Bayles, Michael D (1981) *Professional Ethics*, Wadsworth, Belmont.

Bowles, Wendy, Collingridge, Michael, Curry, Steven and Valentine, Bruce (2006) *Ethical Practice in Social Work*, Allen & Unwin, Sydney.

Davis, Michael (2002) *Profession, Code and Ethics*, Ashgate, Aldershot.

Harris, John (1980) *Violence and Responsibility*, Routledge & Kegan Paul, London, p 128.

Ibsen, Henrik (1961) *A Doll's House*, Oxford, London, Act III, pp 282–83.

Miller, Seumas (2001) 'Ch 8: Collective responsibility' in Miller, Seumas (2001) *Social Action: A Teleological Account*, Cambridge University Press, New York.

— (2006) 'Collective moral responsibility' in French, Peter and Wettstein, Howard (eds) *Midwest Studies in Philosophy*, vol 30, pp 176–93.

— (2009) *The Moral Foundations of Social Institutions: A Philosophical Study*, Cambridge University Press, New York.

Sartre, Jean-Paul (1956) *Being and Nothingness*, Philosophical Library, New York, Pt 1, Ch 2, p 59.

Walzer, Michael (1984) *Just and Unjust Wars*, Penguin, Harmondsworth, pp 141–42.

7: Duty of care, autonomy, paternalism and informed consent

In 1932, the United States Public Health Service (USPHS) initiated the Tuskegee Syphilis Study to document the natural history of syphilis. The subjects of the investigation were 399 poor black sharecroppers from Macon County, Alabama, with latent syphilis and 201 men without the disease who served as controls. The physicians conducting the Study deceived the men, telling them that they were being treated for 'bad blood'. However, they deliberately denied treatment to the men with syphilis and they went to extreme lengths to ensure that they would not receive therapy from any other sources. In exchange for their participation, the men received free meals, free medical examinations, and burial insurance.

It is clear that the US government scientists irreparably harmed hundreds of socially and economically vulnerable African-American men in Macon County, their family members, and their descendants by deliberately deceiving them and withholding from them state of the art treatment. When the Tuskegee Study began, the standard therapy for syphilis consisted of painful injections of arsenical compounds, supplemented by topical applications of mercury or bismuth ointments. Although this therapy was less effective than penicillin would prove to be, in the 1930s every major textbook on syphilis recommended it for the treatment of the disease. After penicillin became available, the researchers withheld its use as well. Published medical reports have estimated that between 28 and 100 men died as a result of their syphilis. Due to a lax study protocol, we cannot be sure that all the men had latent syphilis. It is therefore entirely possible that the infected men passed syphilis to their sexual partners and to their children in utero. Thus the physical harm may not be limited just to the men enrolled in the Study.

Final Report of the Tuskegee Syphilis Study Legacy Committee, 20 May 1996

CASE STUDY 7.2

The Gulf war was the most toxic battle in western military history. We exposed our own troops to major toxins. When I became chief scientific advisor to the British Gulf war veterans, I naïvely expected their health problems to be handled with integrity by the authorities. Instead I came up against corrupt politics, bad medicine and science prostituted in the service of the military.

My involvement with the veterans' fight for medical help from the Ministry of Defence (MoD) began in 1997. I became their representative on the supposedly independent panel for the assessment of government research on the possible interaction between the vaccines and Naps [anti-nerve gas tablets].

Veterans regard the combination of vaccines and Naps tablets as the major causes of their illnesses. Some needed immediate hospital treatment as a result of adverse reactions.

Many report having jabs for smallpox, botulism plague, which never appeared on their notes. Medical records have been 'misplaced'. But there is enough information to show that large numbers of vaccines were given together and in breach of safety guidelines.

The anthrax vaccine administered only protected troops against six of the 22 strains which might have been used by Saddam. They had no warning of exposure to other biological and chemical agents liberated when Iraqi ammunition dumps were blown up in March 1991 because vital monitoring equipment was switched off.

Exposure to these agents, thought to include Sarin and VX nerve gas, can be linked directly to the chronic illnesses suffered by veterans are experiencing, including multiple organ damage.

US and UK forces also fired 630000lbs of depleted uranium-tipped armour-piercing shells at Iraqi targets. Depleted uranium (DU) is an extremely toxic heavy metal and the allied bombing distributed at least 300 tonnes of DU dust over much of the battlefield.

Inhalation of these fine particles damages the kidneys, the immune system and the nervous system. There is also an increased risk of lymphatic cancer as it collects in the bone. Pentagon documents reveal that the US military was aware of these risks decades ago. But the MoD continues to disregard this evidence.

Malcolm Hooper (2003) 'The Gulf War was the most toxic battle in Western military history' *The Guardian*, 4 February

CASE STUDY 7.3

Finally, I reach the issue of surgical culture, which might be a little controversial. How do doctors make clinical-practice decisions? I started with this question to myself on a particular day in an operating theatre somewhere in Australia, where I anaesthetised a woman undergoing hysterectomy because she had depression. Then I followed up by anaesthetising a woman for an endometrial ablation, and who the consultant gynaecologist actually said would be far better treated with a Levonogestrel IUD, but it was good practice for the Registrar.

In 1980, Professor Scully wrote an ethnography of the behaviour of two institutions, one a private and one a public provider of obstetric care, nearly 20 years later Dr Pearl Katz did a similar study of an 800 bed surgical hospital in Canada, where she looked at the behaviour of a group of general surgeons. Both these studies talked of a surgical culture where the prime priority is the mastery of technical skills and the development of a self-assurance in the face of any problem which tended to make it difficult to consult with other colleagues and to back down from decisions made. Both studies found the development of the surgeons' distance from their patients in an attempt to hold up the myth of the doctor as scientist and objective decision-maker. With the development of this surgical culture arises the theory of organization deviance where an entire organization condones, and even nurtures behaviour that would not be acceptable in general society. Members of this culture then justify the reasons for their decisions, trying to bring their *ad hoc* decisions in line with the myth of being scientific, evidence-based medicine providers.

Alison Lilley (2001) 'Hysterectomy service variations – provider behaviour', Paper given at the Women's Health Victoria's Forum, 2 July

CASE STUDY 7.4

A California case illustrates that a patient who declines ECT after receiving information mandated by statute is not necessarily incapable of giving informed consent to such an intervention. In that instance, a conservator had been appointed when it was found that the patient was incapable of providing for his essential personal needs. He had a long-standing history of mental illness for which he had been receiving lithium. His condition was relatively stable until the medication was discontinued due to its side effects. He then became severely psychotic and was hospitalised with a diagnosis of 'schizo-affective illness, excited phase.' Several ECT hearings were held and subsequently ECT was administered. On appeal, the court pointed out that while the patient was extremely psychotic and experienced delusional fears, his psychotic state of mind was intermittent. He appreciated that ECT was proposed to help him. However, having heard the possible effects and side effects of the treatment, the patient believed that it would scramble his brain and kill him. Indeed, he became agitated and psychotic when doctors tried to discuss the treatment with him. At a hearing on his refusal to authorise ECT, the patient was responsive and he followed a logical series of questions and answers. As the appellate court noted, this evidenced a coherent train of thought. The man having experienced ECT before, now feared he could die from it and he felt he could get better with medications.

On appeal, the court determined that there was no evidence that the patient could not appreciate and act intelligently upon the information required to be disclosed under California state law. He had both a psychotic and rational fear of ECT that caused him to refuse consent to such treatment. The court concluded that the record was absent of any clear and convincing evidence to support the finding of incapacity to give informed consent.

Fay A Rozovsky (1990) Consent to Treatment: A Practical Guide

CASE STUDY 7.5

Allegations that the troubled Alder Hey hospital in Liverpool sold human tissue to a French drug company for use in one of its profit-making products yesterday caused a further public outcry over the apparently cavalier attitude of the medical profession to patients' bodies.

Just days before the publication of a report on the removal and storage of hundreds of children's organs at Alder Hey without parents' knowledge, it emerged that supplies of the thymus gland, which is routinely removed during cardiac surgery to give better access to the heart, were regularly handed over to the pharmaceutical company Aventis Pasteur, in exchange for cash donations to the hospital.

The tiny glands were used in the manufacture of a drug for aplastic anaemia.

Alder Hey parents yesterday expressed their horror at the idea of money changing hands for body parts, no matter what the hospital's motivation might have been. They said they were appalled that the hospital would hand over human tissue without the explicit consent of the patients' parent or guardian.

'This brings us right back to the issue of openness and informed consent', said Ed Bradley of the support group Pity II. 'Pity II is not against research. But the hospital has ignored the families and not taken them into account at all.'

Had they been asked, he said, the parents would probably have agreed to the use of the tissue.

Ministers, alarmed at yet another escalation of the Alder Hey crisis, moved swiftly to condemn any exchange of cash for organs. 'This is yet another piece of deeply distressing news for the parents of children treated at Alder Hey', the health secretary, Alan Milburn, said. However, he took pains to point out that, according to the hospital, it happened between 1991 and 1993, then stopped because of concerns among staff that accepting donations for organs might be unethical.

'This was a particular practice which was happening in the early 90s at Alder Hey and, it seems, some other hospitals', he said. 'The NHS already knows this practice of taking organs without consent is totally unacceptable to this government.'

The government would issue further guidance to the NHS, he said, hinting that it would form part of their response to the Alder Hey report, which is published next Tuesday.

Sarah Boseley and David Ward (2001) 'Cash for tissue revelations add to trials of children's hospital', *The Guardian*, 27 January

CASE STUDY 7.6

Baby Fae was born on October 12, 1984, suffering from hypoplastic left heart syndrome, a condition where the left side of the heart is too weak to pump blood. The result is usually death. There was a surgical procedure available at the time called the Norwood Procedure that had a forty percent rate of success when performed by its originator, Dr William Norwood. Heart transplantation was also a possible treatment for this condition. Even when the Norwood Procedure was not totally successful, it could extend a child's life long enough to find a human heart. In the Baby Fae case, however, Dr Leonard Bailey proposed performing a xenograft in which he would transplant a heart from a baboon to the child. The parents agreed to this. Nine days after the procedure Dr Bailey predicted that Baby Fae might celebrate her twentieth birthday. Baby Fae died eleven days later. Commentators questioned whether he had adequately informed the parents about the Norwood Procedure. It appears that a newborn heart was available for transplantation but that Dr Bailey did not look for a donor heart. Also, the consent form he used was inadequate and possibly misleading. For example, the consent form stated that seven years' experience with heart transplants in 150 newborn animals 'suggests that long term survival with appropriate growth and development may be possible …' It does not note, however, that every attempt to use a xenograft in humans has failed.

Leonard H Glantz (1994) 'The law of human experimentation
with children'

CASE STUDY 7.7

Mrs Whitaker underwent elective eye surgery to her blind right eye; she was a curious patient and asked numerous questions to clarify her concerns regarding her vision in her 'good' left eye; and Dr Rogers failed to warn Mrs Whitaker of the remote risk (a 1 in 14 000 chance) of total blindness.

The High Court found that Dr Rogers breached his duty of care to Mrs Whitaker because she was not fully warned of the risks associated with the procedure.

In terms of consent, the Court's summarised findings were:

- consent is valid once a patient is informed in broad terms of the nature of a given procedure;
- adequacy of information depends on the patient's apprehended capacity to understand;
- therapeutic privilege is only permitted in limited circumstances; and
- a patient's desire for information is relevant.

Health and Community Services Complaints Commission
'Informed Consent'

Beverley Matthews, 33, of Stockport, Greater Manchester, was suffering from toxic shock syndrome when she was taken to Stepping Hill hospital with chronic sickness and diarrhoea.

She failed to respond to antibiotics and her condition deteriorated rapidly. Hospital consultants told her that she would have a 30% chance of survival if she had a blood transfusion, but she and her family refused. Mrs Matthews died several hours later.

The coroner, John Pollard ... said the consultant had been blunt enough to say death was inevitable, but Mrs Matthews and her family had refused treatment. He added that her condition was so serious that a transfusion may not have saved her.

Mrs Matthews was the mother of a four-year-old son, Jake, and lived with her husband, Ian, in Bredbury, Stockport. Her family had been Jehovah's Witnesses for 25 years, although her husband is not thought to share her beliefs.

Mrs Matthews's mother, Marie Vernon, said: 'I was looking for the truth and this religion gave me that. She made the right decision – she had to stick to her beliefs. Beverley was a lovely girl.'

Jehovah's Witnesses base their beliefs on three passages in the Bible which order them to abstain from blood.

Derek Casey, a spokesman for the Jehovah's Witnesses, said: 'Jehovah's Witnesses' love of life moves them to seek the best medical treatment for themselves and their families. However, they respect and obey the plain scriptural command to abstain from blood.'

'She loved life and in harmony with her religious beliefs, chose non-blood medical management of her condition.'

Helen Carter (2000) 'Jehovah's witness died after refusing transfusion', *The Guardian*, 20 January

Differences in opinion over the best treatment for [carcinoma in situ, CIS] were one thing. There was always unanimity in the medical community about the object of treatment – to return to a negative or normal smear. A positive smear was a sign that treatment had not been successful; there was still disease present and there had been no 'cure'. In such cases, further treatment was called for, until the smear became normal.

This was never the intention with the National Women's Hospital experiment. Some women with evidence of disease were to be left. They would be followed – that is, brought back for regular smears and possibly more biopsies – but there was no intention to cure them.

But by watching these women, Green hoped to observe the natural history of the disease and prove his thesis that untreated CIS rarely if at all led to invasion.

Green was out on a limb … He called others' belief in progression a 'dogma' which had become 'almost unchallengeable' and so he set about challenging it …

In answer to a question from us about whether women were told there were differences of opinion about the methods of treatment, Green replied: 'I suppose not.' In answer to the same question, Professor Bonham said: 'I wouldn't know, you would have to ask each individual doctor who treated patients.'

Although the HMC, which passed the study, acted as an ethical committee, there was no hospital plan to seek the agreement of the women to their unorthodox management. Consequently, patients like Claire Matheson did not know they were being studied, nor that they were being treated in an unorthodox way.

Sandra Coney (1988) *The Unfortunate Experiment*

CASE STUDY 7.10

Jenny is a 14-year-old girl staying at a youth refuge in the inner city. She has been homeless for about two years and lives either on the streets or in various youth refuges and shelters. She has a drug problem and is a prostitute from time to time. One day Jenny comes to see the social worker Bill, at the refuge. Bill has been a social worker with youth for several years, though he has only been at the refuge for a few months.

Jenny tells Bill that Geoffrey, the new manager at the refuge, was at the last refuge where she stayed. She claims that Geoffrey was sacked from his previous position due to allegations of sexual abuse of girls at the refuge. 'Now he wants to see me in his office, saying I'm in trouble' she says. 'I don't want to see him alone. Will you come with me?'

Bill knows that Geoffrey often has interviews in his office with the door closed, with clients of the refuge. He also knows that Jenny has a reputation for tall stories and troublemaking and has been expelled from other refuges in the area for sexually promiscuous behaviour.

Provided by Wendy Bowles

CASE STUDY 7.11

Stanley Milgram conducted a research study in 1963 on blind obedience to authority in order to better understand the power of the Nazis in Germany. In a psychology laboratory at Yale University, Milgram had volunteers placed in the situation where on his command they were to administer electric shocks that ranged up to 450 volts to other supposed 'volunteers'. 450 volts is sufficient to kill a person. Unbeknown to the volunteers whose role was to administer the shocks, the persons supposedly receiving the shocks were in fact confederates working with Milgram, and in fact were not receiving any electric shocks. It was a case of deception set up for the purpose of observing the extent of the volunteers' blind obedience to an authority figure, viz Milgram. Two-thirds of the volunteers submitted to Milgram's commands and 'administered' the shocks, or at least believed that they had. These people cried and pleaded with Milgram to let them stop. Subsequent to the experiment when these volunteers discovered they had been deceived they were very upset and deeply ashamed.

Provided by the authors

Umberto is lying in the intensive care unit of the hospital after intentionally driving his car into a tree in order to kill himself. He formed an intention to kill himself after his de facto, Kirrilly, finally terminated their relationship. They had been living apart for two weeks. Umberto is brain dead, though 'life support' systems are enabling the ongoing functioning of his heart, lungs and other organs with a view to organ donation and transplantation. Umberto and Kirrilly have a child. Umberto has a mother, Marie, and a father, Pedro. Umberto has given consent for the donation and transplantation of his organs after his death. He did so in order to help other people live longer and better lives. Kirrilly is known to favour the donation of Umberto's organs, since it can help someone else to live a longer and better life. Pedro and Marie are opposed to donating and selling Umberto's body parts. They regard the removal of organs as profoundly disrespectful to the dead. Umberto has $20000 in the bank, but made no will. Kirrilly is on social security.

Provided by the authors

ETHICAL ANALYSIS

Duty of care

The notion of a 'duty of care' is central in professional ethics, especially for human service professionals, like doctors, lawyers and social workers. Duty of care is founded on a very simple and general principle: that each of us should take care not to act in ways which a reasonable person could foresee might harm others. It has also taken on complexities that are important to understand (Jaffey 1992). Before we launch into the complexities, we will first briefly explore the concept of a duty.

Any duty involves a relationship between two (or more) people, the person who has the duty to provide some thing or service, and person to whom they owe the duty. In turn the person to whom the duty is owed can be said to have a right against the first person to demand that thing. Furthermore, if the person who has a duty to supply a thing does not do so, they become liable to sanction for their failure.

Some duties (and hence the corresponding rights) are very specific in terms of the actions that must be undertaken to conform to them. A tenant, for example may have a duty to pay their landlord a hundred dollars every Friday. Other duties are non-specific; they depend on the particular situations in which they apply. Parents, for example, have a duty to foster the physical and emotional wellbeing of their child. But what counts as doing this satisfactorily may vary from family to family and child to child. Sometimes it involves providing music lessons for a child, at other times, helping a child overcome their crippling shyness.

As it has come to be understood in legal and ethical contexts the duty of care is non-specific in two ways, both of which depend on the notion of 'reasonably foreseeable'. Firstly, the duty does not comprehensively detail what we must do. Clearly, we must not do things that are likely to harm others *directly and immediately*. We should not, for example, throw boiling water from an upper-storey window without checking that it is safe to do so. But we are also required not to act in ways that could be reasonably foreseen to create risks of future harm to others, and to get rid of those risks if we have created them. Hence, according to the legal doctrine of 'attractive nuisances', a person who owns a trampoline which can be accessed by neighbourhood children has a duty to either make it safe for their use or block their access.

Thus, which actions we should take to satisfy our duty of care will be matters of judgment. A landlord, for example, who has been warned that the electrical wiring in a house he is renting is in an unsafe condition, is required by his duty of care to replace it. Another landlord, who has been informed by an electrician that the wiring in the house he lets out is sound, has acted in accordance with his duty of care, even if it turns out that it is actually unsafe and the house burns down as a result.

The duty of care is also non-specific in terms of who the recipient of the duty is (in other words, who has a right not to be harmed). The landlord, for example, whose rental property burns down after he has been warned that the electrical wiring is unsafe, has clearly failed in his duty of care to his tenants. But if the fire spreads, and damages neighbouring properties, he may also be held to have failed in his duty of care to residents and owners of those properties.

Duties of care, nevertheless, are not completely open-ended. Firstly, many of our activities by their very nature impose risks on others (driving a car or undertaking surgery). Given that these activities are seen as legitimate, and even necessary, it would be unreasonable to interpret the duty of care so stringently that we could not undertake them. That would mean, for example, no-one would drive on freeways, due to the risk of accidents. (While we shouldn't simply stop taking such risks, we still need to take due care when undertaking these activities.)

Secondly, the consequences of our actions can ripple out from us in unpredictable ways and harm people far removed from us. However, since we cannot reasonably foresee these specific harms, the duty of care does not forbid us from acting in ways that create a risk of such distant harm. Indeed, a constitutive feature of the duty of care is that we can only have such a duty to someone with whom we are in what the law calls a 'proximate relationship'. The most obvious example of such a relationship is one of spatial closeness, as the term implies. But there are other ways of entering such a relationship.

In particular members of certain occupational groups – notably professional groups – come to have duties of care to those they serve and in some ways these duties can be more stringent and extensive than those that apply to us in our ordinary life. As we saw in Chapter 6, our collective moral responsibilities to assist one another have given rise to specialised roles to better facilitate the provision of such assistance. These roles include that of doctor, nurse, social worker, police officer, fireman, accountant, teacher, and so on.

In virtue of accepting someone as a client (as in the case of a doctor or nurse), or taking on a role dedicated to helping anyone who needs it (as in the case of a police officer or fireman), the role occupant has entered into the kind of 'proximate relationship' which is a precondition for the existence of a duty of care. There is a relationship of reliance, indeed trust, between the role occupant and the client or other person to whom the role occupant provides assistance. Having become ill, for example, a person trusts the nurse and doctor to provide health services. Since the role holder has, in effect, asserted their competence in undertaking the role, they are assumed to be able to reasonably foresee the dangers associated with their role-related actions to the level that is appropriate to a competent practitioner.

Moreover, even when the 'client' is an unwilling recipient of services, such as in the case of the mentally ill or of prisoners, providers still owe a special duty of care. This is because the provider of the 'service' has taken over certain responsibilities that formerly attached, or ordinarily attach, to the persons themselves. For example, once imprisoned an inmate cannot provide food for themselves, and may be at great risk from other dangerous inmates. Accordingly, correctional staff have a duty of care to inmates to ensure that the prisoners are properly fed, kept safe, and so on.

Those who employ, or are otherwise in authority, also have a duty of care in relation to employees or other subordinates who have entrusted aspects of their welfare to the organisation in question. Case studies 7.1 and 7.2 illustrate the failure to discharge the moral and (typically) legal duty of care on the part of a health service and a defence force (respectively).

A key feature of the relationship between members of the professions and other related occupational groups is the vulnerability of many of their clients. They lack the knowledge, skill and so on to achieve their desired ends, and rely on professionals to assist them in doing so. The power of the practitioner relative to the client gives rise to the opportunity to abuse that vulnerability and indeed, on occasion, to a culture of such abuse. (See case studies 7.1, 7.3, 7.6, 7.9, 7.10 and 7.11.) Such abuse, it goes without saying, is completely morally unacceptable. But the duty of a professional to their client goes further than simply not abusing them and helping them. The *way* in which professionals assist their clients is also morally significant. In particular, professionals ought to act in ways that respect and promote their clients' autonomy. We look to some of the implications of this below in our discussions of informed consent and paternalism, but to do justice to these concepts we must first focus on the nature of autonomy itself.

Autonomy

The word 'autonomy' derives from the two Greek words '*auto*' ('self') and '*nomos*' ('law'). The term was originally applied to states: an autonomous state was one that laid down its own laws, rather than having them imposed on it by some outside authority. Similarly, an autonomous person is someone who is able to make well-founded decisions for themselves about how they should act, and to act according to those decisions.

An autonomous person, we argue, is both rational and moral (Miller 2005). Roughly speaking, to call someone rational is to imply that they:

- are possessed of a continuing, integrated structure of mental attitudes, such as beliefs and desires;
- engage in practical (action oriented) and theoretical (knowledge oriented) reasoning that makes use of objectively valid procedures, such as deriving valid conclusions from evidence; and
- are disposed to make true judgments and valid inferences in so doing.

Moreover, a rational person is disposed to intentionally act on the judgments that result from their practical reasoning. Further, since people have finite lives, and know this, rational people make their plans – including their life plan – accordingly. Rationality in this sense admits of degrees; some people, for example, are better than others at drawing true conclusions from the evidence presented to them.

Someone can be rational, up to a point, without necessarily being moral. They may, for example, be capable of developing and putting into practices plans to get things they want, without caring if others are hurt in the process. However, people operate in an interpersonal and social world, in which moral reasons abound. Someone who does not recognise those reasons, or does not respond to them in the right way, is not simply less than fully moral, they are also less than fully rational. Roughly speaking, a human moral agent is a rational agent who is disposed to make true judgments and valid inferences in relation to the moral worth of human actions, attitudes, motivations, emotions, agents, and so on, and to act on those judgments and inferences where appropriate.

Here it is worth noting the distinction between non-rational and irrational agents, and between non-moral and immoral agents. A non-rational agent *cannot* make judgments or inferences. An irrational agent has the capacity to make such judgments and inferences, but has some significant deficit in their rationality, and thus makes a significant number of false judgments and/or invalid inferences, or often fails to act on the results of their practical reasoning. Similarly, a non-moral agent lacks the capacity to make moral judgments and act on them; an immoral agent, by contrast, is merely (significantly) deficient in their moral judgment-making or often fails to act on their correct moral judgments. That said, sometimes it is not clear whether we should think of a person as non-moral (or non-rational) or as immoral (or irrational). (See case study 7.4.)

Given that a fully human life involves responsiveness to moral reasons, an autonomous person will thus be both rational and moral. Understood in the way outlined here, rationality and morality imply independence and self-mastery. Someone who is dominated by the overriding desire to please an authority figure, and who only acts in accordance with that aim, will not count as autonomous. This is true even if the authority figure themselves is a highly reliable guide to prudent action and true belief, and even if the person who aims to please them knows this. Independence from undue reliance on others, then, is a necessary condition for autonomy. (At the same time, complete isolation from, or mistrust, of others, actually reduces autonomy, since it cuts us off from sources of advice, guidance and so on that are likely to make us better able to identify and respond to reasons.) Similarly, the autonomous person must be able not only to make good judgments about what to believe and how to act, they must be capable of acting in conformity with those judgments. A drug addict, for example, may know perfectly well that it is unwise to keep feeding their addiction, but find themselves unable to act on that knowledge; their lack of self-mastery in respect of their desire for the drug means that they lack autonomy, at least in this area of their life.

To say that an autonomous person is independent and possesses self-mastery, does not, of course, imply that autonomy is incompatible with all forms of constraint. The autonomous person cannot infringe the laws of physics or the laws of logic. The fact that a human agent cannot hope to fly when they jump off a tall building, or cannot both walk and not walk at the same time, does not undermine their autonomy. And there are other constraints on human agents which do not undermine their autonomy. Some of these are generated by psycho-physiological features of humans. Consider the inability of humans to freely determine what their perceptual and bodily sensations will be, or the inability of most humans to withstand the pain of extreme torture for long periods. Other constraints are generated by psycho-moral features, such as the basic desire to be approved of by at least some other human beings, and the basic disposition to approve of oneself. We assume that these logical, physical and psychological constraints are just that: constraints. As such, they constrain what a human agent can be, and what they can do; but they do not necessarily fully determine what such an agent is or does. So autonomy is not ruled out by the existence of such constraints.

It follows from our discussion that the adjective 'autonomous' applies in the first instance to individual people, and derivatively to the choices that such people make or the lives that they lead. When we talk about a person being autonomous, we mean that they can decide for themselves what is important and valuable to them, and possess the capacity to make reason-based choices on the basis of recognising, assessing and responding to relevant facts, including moral facts. When we call an act autonomous, we mean that it is something done by such a person, on the basis of such a response. When we call a life autonomous, we mean that it is lived by an autonomous person and that it provides sufficient opportunity for the making of autonomous choices. Autonomy thus contrasts with at least some notions of freedom, like expressions such as 'a freely performed action'. It does not make much sense to say that John was an autonomous agent for 10 seconds of his life, or that some action was autonomously performed, even though the agent who performed it lacked autonomy.

It also follows that autonomy admits of degree. None of us, presumably, is completely autonomous, since we all fall short of full rationality, perfect morality, absolute self-mastery and so on. And since these things vary from person to person, some people are more autonomous than others. Moreover, someone might be autonomous in one area of their life, but not another. (See case study 7.4.) Nevertheless, we achieve the status of an autonomous person – someone who is entitled to decide for themselves how they wish to live – when we are sufficiently autonomous. There is a presumption that all adults, at least, have achieved that status. This presumption is defeasible. We may be able to show that a person is so deficient in various conditions of autonomy, such as rationality or self-mastery, that they should not be counted as autonomous, and that others might be justified in making decisions on their behalf. But absent such defeat, we all possess the status of autonomous persons.

Paternalism

Paternalism involves one person acting to make something happen to another, or forcing the other to act, or preventing them from acting, for the good of that person, but despite or irrespective of the wishes of the other. Paternalism, as its name implies, is to be understood by analogy with the relationship between a father and his young child. The father is often justified in imposing his will on the child for the child's own good: to make them go to school when they don't want to, or to stop them eating more junk food, and so on. That kind of behaviour may be justified when it is directed to a child who does not, or cannot, understand the consequences of their action. As adults, of course, we resent having our wishes overridden by others in matters that concern us, even if such action is motivated by concern for our wellbeing and the desire to help us. Our resentment reflects the fact that the paternalist treats us as less than fully autonomous. We are likely to feel this resentment even when, as it happens, we were wrong about what was in our interests and the person who acted paternalistically towards us was correct. After all, we have, so to speak, a 'right to be wrong'; and others have no right to impose their will on us in matters that are our business.

So, generally, paternalism is morally offensive, at least when directed to autonomous individuals, and to be avoided; generally, but perhaps not always. To understand why paternalism might occasionally be justified we need to consider the distinction between so-called 'soft' and 'hard' paternalism (Dworkin 1988). To illustrate soft paternalism, consider the following kind of situation. We see a pedestrian about to cross a footbridge whose foundations we know have been dangerously undermined by overnight flooding. As we begin to explain the danger the pedestrian impatiently tries to brush past us to walk onto the bridge. To prevent them from doing so we place our body across the narrow entrance.

This is an example of soft paternalism. Soft paternalism involves one person acting to make something happen to another, or forcing the other to act, or preventing them from acting, for the good of that person, but despite or irrespective of the wishes of the other, *where the wishes of the other reflect a lack of full autonomy*. In the bridge case, even though the pedestrian is (we are assuming) an autonomous person, their *decision* was not fully autonomous, since they lacked vital information on which to base it. (Recall the distinction made in the section on autonomy between an autonomous person and an autonomous act.)

Most people will think soft paternalism is justified in this case. We can generalise.

(Soft) paternalism may be justified where the following conditions apply:

1) the person to whom the paternalistic act is directed is otherwise likely to act (or fail to act) in ways that will have severe harmful (and especially irreversible) consequences;
2) that person is (probably) not aware of the consequences of their actions, or their ability to appreciate those consequences is impaired (through drugs, passion, mental illness etc);
3) the paternalist is able to see and avert these consequences, and has good reason to believe that conditions 1) and 2) apply;
4) there is no feasible way of putting the person to whom the paternalistic act is to be directed in a position to make an autonomous decision (through, for example, providing them with relevant information, helping them overcome the passion which is clouding their judgment etc).

Hard paternalism involves acting paternalistically even where the decision of the (autonomous) person towards whom we are acting paternalistically is itself autonomous. Imagine, to continue our story about the pedestrian, that after we manage to convey to him the dangers of walking on the bridge, he tells us that this makes the bridge all the more attractive to him, since he is a thrillseeker, constantly looking for dangerous challenges. If we still prevented him from going onto the bridge, we would be hard paternalists.

Hard paternalism is obviously much more problematic than soft paternalism, since it involves one person deliberately overriding another's autonomous decision. Even so, it is a morally complex phenomenon. On the one hand, the paternalist is motivated by the desire to help the person to whom their paternalistic act is directed, and the motivation to help others is in itself morally good. On the other hand, the hard paternalist will act irrespective of, or even against, the autonomous wishes of the person they are trying to help. In as much as this involves disregarding or overriding another person's autonomy, it is morally bad. Hard paternalism, it seems, involves a conflict between two very basic moral principles: beneficence (help others), and respect for autonomy.

As we pointed out in the early chapters of this book, we do not accept that there is any ranking of moral principles such that when two principles clash, one must always prevail over the other. So it is at least conceivable that beneficence might on very rare occasions trump respect for autonomy and that, therefore, hard paternalism be justified. There will however be few, if any, such cases in practice, given the importance of the principle of respect for autonomy and, in particular, given the strong presumption that a person possessed of autonomy is the best judge of what is good for him or herself.

Paternalism (both soft and hard) presents particular moral challenges – and temptations – in many professional settings. Firstly, beneficence is a weighty value for professionals in their dealings with their clients. Since professionals have taken on an obligation to their clients, it is not simply that it would be good if they helped them, but they must try to do so. Moreover, it is not uncommon for clients to be unwilling or unable to act in the way that the professional judges to be in their best interests, even though the professional may often be in a much better position to know what is in the client's interest, at least within their area of professional expertise, than the client. Finally, clients themselves, particularly those who are facing major life-choices regarding their health or their freedom, may actually prefer not to take responsibility for their decisions, and to allow professionals to make decisions on their behalf.

For reasons pointed to above, generally professionals (like everyone else) should avoid hard paternalism. However, again as noted above, there might be exceptions. Consider in this context case study 7.8 in which for religious reasons Beverley Matthews refused a blood transfusion, even though the doctor told her that she would die without it. If the doctor had transfused without her permission her survival would have been more likely. However, it is not necessarily wrong not to help a person stay alive, especially if doing so would offend a value central to that person's self-understanding. In Beverley's view it was more important for her to live – and die – in a way that was consistent with her deep religious convictions than to accept the transfusion. Understood in this way she is exercising her autonomy, notwithstanding that she will (in effect) kill herself in so doing. However, it is far from clear that the doctor should not intervene to save her and, thereby, act in accordance with the principle of hard paternalism. It might be argued that the value of life here outweighs the value of autonomy.

On the other hand, it might be argued that even if the doctor gave her the blood transfusion he would not necessarily be overriding her autonomy; for it might be claimed she is not morally autonomous. The problem here is the irrational nature of her specific religiously-based moral belief in relation to blood transfusion. It is a false belief both with respect to:

- content (it is false that refusing a blood transfusion is a moral requirement); and

- moral importance (even if it were a moral requirement in some circumstances it could not be a requirement of such moral weight as to override the value of life itself).

A person who acts on such false moral beliefs is not necessarily to be ascribed moral autonomy.

Since soft paternalism might on occasion be justified, there may be times when professionals can justifiably act in a soft paternalistic way towards their clients. Psychiatrists may, for example, be justified in committing clients who are having a psychotic episode to an institution against their will, at least until they are able to respond to reason again.

Professionals should, however, be wary of too glib recourse to paternalistic action. Recall that the fourth of the conditions above for justifying a soft paternalistic action is that there is no way of putting the person in a position to make an autonomous decision. (Through, for example, providing them with relevant information, helping them overcome the passion which is clouding their judgment etc.) But of course often, in dealings between professionals and clients, there is such a way. The recognition of this possibility has led in recent decades to the emphasis on informed consent.

Informed consent

Like duty of care, the notion of informed consent is based on a simple idea: that we should not interfere with people who can decide for themselves unless they have consented to our doing so. This is, of course, an implication of respect for autonomy. As paternalistic attitudes and practices have come to be seen as unacceptable in professional practice over the past few decades, informed consent has taken on legal and ethical complexities; again, like duty of care (Faden and Beauchamp 1986). Indeed, the two notions are closely tied, since one way a professional in particular can fail in their duty of care is by not gaining informed consent to engage in some action which impacts on their client (Rozovsky 1990).

Case study 7.11 (the Milgram experiment) describes a situation where the subjects did not consent to what was done to them. Indeed, they could not have consented, since the experiment depended on their believing that they were actually harming others, when they were not. The subjects were simply used by the experimenters to test a hypothesis. Such action is in direct conflict with respect for autonomy, and for this reason any such experiment would now be forbidden.

In many of the activities we undertake, our informed consent can reasonably be assumed. Any adult surely understands that they are likely to be frightened if they go on a roller-coaster ride. Their consent to being frightened can be assumed from their willingness to take the ride.

Informed consent becomes more important, and complicated, when, while it is possible that those affected by some action could consent (unlike the Milgram case), such consent cannot simply be assumed. Consider here the situation described in case study 7.5 where parts were taken from the bodies of children who had died at Alder Hey hospital. According to a spokesperson for the parents, 'Had they been asked ... the parents would probably have agreed to use of the tissue.' But obviously in a case involving such sensitive issues, there could be no general assumption of consent. Furthermore, there is a fundamental difference in such cases between acting in a way that would have been consented to by those affected if they had been asked, and actually obtaining such consent.

Where consent cannot simply be assumed, the conditions for a person giving informed consent are that the person:

- is competent to give consent;
- is properly informed about the course of action;
- makes a valid expression of consent.

Let us consider these conditions in turn. Competence, in the sense in which it is used here, is very similar to rationality, as we defined it in our discussion of autonomy above. That is, the competent person not only has the capacity to seek out and understand information presented to them, and to draw valid conclusions from such information, but must have a continuing, integrated structure of mental attitudes, such as beliefs and desires. To see the importance of the possession of such a mental structure, think of a person who is contemplating undergoing extensive plastic surgery in order to improve their chances of pursuing a successful career as an actor. Whether this person has a settled, considered ambition to follow an acting career, or is incapable of settling on any long-term goals and is merely acting on a whim, will make a large difference as to whether it is reasonable for them to be exposed to the dangers of major surgery.

We should note that just as autonomy and rationality can be relativised to particular areas of one's life, so can competence. Consider here case study 7.4 where a mentally ill patient was held competent to consent – or in this case refuse to consent – to electric shock treatment. That this person was not competent in other areas of his life did not mean that he could not understand the implications of accepting or refusing such treatment.

The second condition for informed consent is the possession of the information necessary for a competent person to make a properly informed choice. In technically complex areas, such as medicine or law, we often rely on service providers to provide us with such information. Granted, it will often be impossible for the layperson to have the same level of understanding as the experts. But they can be given information in a form which allows them to understand such things as the possible courses of action available to them, the likely costs, benefits and risks associated with these, as well as the professional's own view of the most desirable course of action.

Different views exist about what a competent person needs to be told so that they can make a properly informed choice. At least, they should be given the information that any reasonable person would need to know. (This is known as the objective test.) In the 'Baby Fae' case, described in case study 7.6, although Fae's parents were (presumably) competent and agreed to their daughter having a transplant of a baboon's heart, that agreement could not count as informed consent. The reason is that they clearly had not been provided with information that any reasonable person would need to know to make an informed decision. In particular, they had not been told about other treatments, and the likelihood of success and failure of the various options.

Arguably, people should also be provided with information that *they* are likely to want to know, even if not every reasonable person would. (This is known as the subjective test.) Consider case study 7.7. Obviously any reasonable person considering undergoing some surgical procedure would want to know about likely serious adverse consequences of such intervention. On the other hand, they may not want to know about very unlikely, but possible, adverse consequences. The risk of going blind as a result of the surgery that Mrs Whitaker underwent was one chance in 14 000: that surely counts as very unlikely. Nevertheless, given the concerns that Mrs Whitaker expressed to her surgeon about that very outcome the court determined that he should have told her of the (remote) risk. He did not, and therefore she was deprived of information that she needed to give informed consent.

Finally, informed consent requires a valid expression of consent (made by a competent, properly informed person). A valid expression of consent will indicate that the person has understood what they are agreeing to, and furthermore is made for the right reasons (not under duress, desperation and so on).

Readings

Boseley, Sarah and Ward, David (2001) 'Cash for tissue revelations add to trials of children's hospital', 27 January, available at <http://www.guardian.co.uk> (accessed 23/1/09).

Carter, Helen (2000) 'Jehovah's witness died after refusing transfusion', *The Guardian*, 20 January, available at <http://www.guardian.co.uk> (accessed 23/1/09).

Christman, John (ed) (1989) *The Inner Citadel: Essays on Individual Autonomy*, Oxford University Press, New York.

Coney, Sandra (1988) *The Unfortunate Experiment*, Penguin, Auckland, pp 54-55.

Dworkin, Gerald (1988) *Theory and Practice of Autonomy*, Cambridge University Press, Cambridge, New York.

— (1972) 'Paternalism', *The Monist*, vol 56, pp 64-84.

Faden, Ruth and Beauchamp, Tom (1986) *History and Theory of Informed Consent*, Oxford University Press, New York.

Feinberg, Joel (1986) *Harm to Self*, Oxford University Press, Oxford.

Final Report of the Tuskegee Syphilis Study Legacy Committee (1996), 20 May, available at <http://www.tuskegee.edu/Global/story.asp?S=1141982> (accessed 23/1/09).

Glantz, Leonard H (1994) 'The law of human experimentation with children' in Grodin, Michael and Glantz, Leonard (eds) *Children as Research Subjects: Science, Ethics and Law*, Oxford University Press, New York, pp 126-27.

Health and Community Services Complaints Commission 'Informed consent', available at <http://www.nt.gov.au/omb_hcscc/hcscc/pdf/informed_consent.pdf> (accessed 23/1/09).

Hooper, Malcolm (2003) 'The Gulf War was the most toxic battle in Western military history', *The Guardian*, 4 February, available at <http://www.guardian.co.uk> (accessed 23/1/09).

Jaffey, Anthony (1992) *The Duty of Care*, Dartmouth Publishing Company, Aldershot & Hants UK, Brookfield.

Kleinig, John (1983) *Paternalism*, Rowman and Littlefield, Totowa.

Lilley, Alison (2001) 'Hysterectomy service variations - provider behaviour', Paper given at the Women's Health Victoria Forum, 2 July, available at <http://www.whv.org.au/health_issues/hysterectomy.htm> (accessed 23/1/09).

Mackenzie, Catriona and Stoljar, Natalie (eds) (2000) *Relational Autonomy: Feminist Perspectives on Autonomy, Agency, and the Social Self*, Oxford University Press, New York.

Mill, John Stuart (1865) *On Liberty*, Longmans, Green, London (any edition).

Miller, Seumas (2005) 'Individual autonomy and sociality' in Schmitt, Fred (ed) *Socializing Metaphysics*, Rowman Littlefield, Oxford, pp 271-74.

Rozovsky, Fay A (1990) *Consent to Treatment: A Practical Guide*, 2nd edition, Little, Brown and Company, Boston, pp 379-80.

8: Privacy and confidentiality

Jim is a 30-year-old man who has made an appointment to see Clive, a social worker at the local community health centre. During the session, Jim tells Clive that he needs to talk a few things out. He has just found out from the local STD clinic that he is HIV positive. Jim is a successful accountant and has been married for two years. In the past he has been bisexual but his wife, family and friends of many years know nothing of this side of his life. 'I'm not really gay you see', he explains to Clive, 'I just had the odd encounter when I was drunk or stoned.'

Jim says that he wants information on how to protect his wife from cross infection but does not want to tell her about his diagnosis. His wife Julie, he says, is a Christian who does not believe in sex before marriage. Jim is adamant that he cannot tell his wife about his past or his current HIV status, saying that she would leave him if she knew, or perhaps suicide herself. Besides, she might be pregnant and is 'all emotional at the moment anyway'. Jim and Julie have been trying to conceive a child for some months. Julie's period is two weeks late, 'but it could be a false alarm. She isn't regular anyway'.

Provided by Wendy Bowles

CASE STUDY 8.2

Doctors and social workers have rejected calls to break patient confidentiality to inform local authorities of all drug addicts with school-age children.

The professions warned that addicts would avoid seeking help, thereby placing their children in greater danger rather than protecting them from harm.

But they fear that powers to control patient information in the new health and social care bill could allow a moralistic health secretary to force them to breach addicts' confidentiality in the future, claiming it was in the public interest.

Their warnings came after Professor Neil McKeganey, head of Glasgow University's centre for drug misuse research, said GPs, social workers and drugs workers needed to breach confidentiality in the interests of children's welfare.

'The risks posed to these children far outweigh the principle of confidentiality', he argued.

The recommendation came as he revealed details of the first comprehensive study into the impact of drug abuse on the children of addicts in the UK. The three-year project interviewed 70 people who had overcome addiction to illegal drugs.

In the report, the Impact of Drug Dependence on Addicts' Children, parents revealed how their addiction had blighted their children's lives. One described stealing their children's clothes to support their habit, while another admitted failing to protect her son from physical abuse by her partner. Others took their children on late-night drug deals or on shoplifting trips. Children also witnessed their parents injecting drugs and accompanied them to police stations when they were arrested.

Prof McKeganey said: 'Addicts said their children were suffering without any agencies' knowledge and schools often do not know, and are not routinely told, that pupils are living with a parent dependent on drugs. By sharing information professionals would be equipped to intervene before a child was seriously hurt.'

The professor estimates that 20 000 children in Scotland alone have a parent who is an addict. 'Sharing information about drug addicted parents would also lead to a more systematic recording of the number of children in danger', he said.

However, guidance from the General Medical Council, which regulates doctors, states that disclosure of personal information without consent may be justified only where failure to do so may expose the patient or others to death or serious harm.

Dr Michael Wilks, chairman of the British Medical Association's ethics committee, said the potential risks posed to addicts' children were not serious enough to breach confidentiality.

'If you're aware through a child that there's an addict in their family and that relative is also your patient then you have some responsibility to assess the child's welfare. However, you're likely to alienate both parent and child if you breach their trust.'

Rob Hutchinson, chairman of the Association of Directors of Social Services' children's and families committee, said: 'Under jointly agreed child protection procedures there is a need for professionals who believe a child or young person to be at risk of significant harm to share that information with appropriate agencies.

'It should not be assumed however that information should be shared simply because the parent has a drug problem. This does not on its own mean that the child is at risk.'

Ian Robinson, deputy director of drug charity Release, warned addicts would avoid seeking help if their confidentiality was compromised. 'There is already a problem with women not accessing services because they're afraid of losing their children.'

David Batty (2001) 'Calls to break addict confidentiality rejected', *The Guardian*, 7 March

Plaintiff's first cause of action, entitled 'Failure to Detain a Dangerous Patient', alleges that on August 20, 1969, Poddar was a voluntary outpatient receiving therapy at Cowell Memorial Hospital. Poddar informed Moore, his therapist, that he was going to kill an unnamed girl, readily identifiable as Tatiana, when she returned home from spending the summer in Brazil. Moore, with the concurrence of Dr Gold, who had initially examined Poddar, and Dr Yandell, assistant to the director of the department of psychiatry, decided that Poddar should be committed for observation in a mental hospital. Moore orally notified Officers Atkinson and Teel of the campus police that he would request commitment. He then sent a letter to Police Chief William Beall requesting the assistance of the police department in securing Poddar's confinement.

Officers Atkinson, Brownrigg, and Halleran took Poddar into custody, but, satisfied that Poddar was rational, released him on his promise to stay away from Tatiana. Powelson, director of the department of psychiatry at Cowell Memorial Hospital, then asked the police to return Moore's letter, directed that all copies of the letter and notes that Moore had taken as therapist be destroyed, and 'ordered no action to place Prosenjit Poddar in 72-hour treatment and evaluation facility.'

Plaintiff's second cause of action entitled 'Failure to Warn On a Dangerous Patient', incorporates the allegations of the first cause of action, but adds the assertion that defendants negligently permitted Poddar to be released from police custody without 'notifying the parents of Tatiana Tarasoff that their daughter was in grave danger from Prosenjit Poddar.' Poddar persuaded Tatiana's brother to share an apartment with him near Tatiana's residence; shortly after her return from Brazil, Poddar went to her residence and killed her.

Tarasoff v Regents of the University of California (1976)
17 Cal 3d 358, Cal SC

The judge didn't really want to send the former nun to jail, but he felt he had no choice. She was adamantly refusing to turn over to the court a file from the rape crisis centre where she worked. That file contained information about a fifteen-year old victim of a rape who'd come in for counselling. The defendant in the rape case wanted the file to prepare his defence, and as the judge ... interpreted the law, he had a right to it. Thus, when it became clear that Margaret 'Peggy' Langhammer, thirty-one, a drop-out from the order of the Sisters of Mercy and executive director of the Rhode Island Rape Crisis Center (RCC) would not budge, he ordered her to jail ...

Her stay in prison was short: one day. When the victim gave her permission for the file to be released, Langhammer surrendered it to the court and was set free.

It's easy to understand and sympathise with the position Langhammer took ... 'Part of the healing process after a rape is just being able to talk about it', Langhammer told the *Phoenix* in an interview. She added that a victim might not seek a counsellor's help if there was a possibility that her most intimate thoughts might one day surface in a courtroom.

Still, it's equally easy to understand why Arthur Donnelly, twenty-five ... wanted and felt he had a right to what the fifteen year old had said about the assault he was charged with. For all he knew, the RCC file might contain evidence that could allow him to clear his name.

Margaret L Rhodes (1986) *Ethical Dilemmas in Social Work Practice*

In December 1995 the Royal Commission into corrupt New South Wales police officers was shown surveillance camera video of Detective Sergeant Wayne Eade, discussing drug deals and the purchase of a child-pornography video with a prostitute, who was also an informer for the Commission.

Royal Commissioner James Wood released copies of the tape (with some bits edited out) to the media and it was shown several times on prime time news and current affairs programs. The officer's family became embroiled in the controversy, even though Wayne Eade had separated from his wife and children some time before the video was shown.

Mrs Susan Eade, and her 16-year-old son, Daniel, appeared on Channel 9's *A Current Affair*, to tell Australia how her life had been ruined by the showing of her disgraced husband's actions. The president of the police union, Phil Tuncheon said many innocent victims would suffer as the result of such scenes being shown on television.

Church groups also condemned the screening of the surveillance camera tapes. A spokesperson for the Catholic Church, Father Brian Lucas, said it was inappropriate to show it when families were watching television. The New South Wales Council of Churches also asked the Royal Commission and television stations to show more restraint.

Commissioner James Wood justified his actions on the grounds of public interest. He also said that showing such material would act as a warning to other corrupt police officers that they could not get away with cheating the public any longer.

An editorial in the tabloid, *Daily Telegraph Mirror*, called for sensitivity in the airing of such video evidence. The *Mirror's* editorial said this is not a question of censorship, but of taste; the editorial also said that the public value of such information was 'dubious'.

However, the *Sydney Morning Herald* editorial supported Justice Wood and the public showing of surveillance material. The editorial said there is an 'obvious sympathy' for Mrs Eade and her family, but that in the end; 'the possibility that corrupt behaviour may be exposed to the world – and their families – may be the best weapon to beat corrupt officers into submission'.

Provided by John Blackler

CASE STUDY 8.6

In 1984 47-year-old Arthur Shelby Lowe, salesman and church elder, was referred to psychotherapist (and former parole officer) Margaret

Hobbs after his arrest for exposing himself to schoolgirls. Lowe was placed by the court on a two-year bond that obliged him to continue therapy with Hobbs. In therapy, Lowe revealed a 30-year history of consistent sexual offending, exposing himself to young women, often exhibiting obscene photographs. The highly experienced Hobbs came to believe that Lowe's problems went much deeper than exhibitionism; furthermore, she did not believe that Lowe was seriously seeking help – indeed, he seemed to gain pleasure from shocking Hobbs with his increasingly sickening revelations.

Lowe's Springvale Court-imposed recognisance expired in 1985, but he continued, on an occasional basis, to consult Hobbs professionally. By 1990, as Hobbs had feared, Lowe's sexual offending was escalating. He told Hobbs he had been interviewed by police, but not charged, after accosting a young girl at Yarraville. Shortly afterwards he was arrested for making sexual remarks and suggestions to girls on Flinders Street Railway Station.

The court imposed a $750 fine; six months later Lowe abducted and murdered six-year-old Sheree Beasley at Rosebud. Hobbs was sure Lowe, who lived in that area, was the abductor.

Over the following months Lowe met with Hobbs over 100 times. It was a gruelling experience for Hobbs, as Lowe obliquely, teasingly began to reveal himself to her as Sheree's killer. On one occasion, after the child's semi-decomposed body had been found, Lowe brought a rucksack containing a plastic bag to Hobbs consulting rooms. In the course of conversation he asked Hobbs with salacious pleasure, 'Margaret, do you really think I could bury a child in a drain to be eaten by maggots?' A mass of maggots were crawling out of Lowe's bag. Hobbs shrieked at Lowe to get out, seized the bag and threw it and its disgusting contents in a bin.

Hobbs was not driven by concern for her client. Unbeknownst to Lowe, Hobbs had established a relationship with the police investigating Sheree Beasley's murder. Supposedly without Hobbs' knowledge the police bugged her Fitzroy consulting rooms. In any case the 'Fitzroy Tapes' became a critical part of the police case against Lowe.

Lowe was arrested and charged with Sheree Beasley's murder in May, 1993.

Provided by the authors

ETHICAL ANALYSIS

In this chapter our primary focus is professional confidentiality, particularly the obligation of confidentiality of professional to client. Confidentiality tends to be given more weight, and to be seen as having wider application, in professional life than in our day-to-day life. Professionals, for example, are held to be obliged to treat as confidential information they gain from or about their clients in their professional dealings, even about things that normally are not seen as matters that need to be kept private. Hence, professional codes of ethics often stress the obligation of professionals to respect confidentiality. Professional confidentiality has a number of moral justifications, depending on the professional settings in question. These justifications include the harm done if confidentiality is breached, the importance of confidentiality as a basis for professional–client trust, and privacy as a moral basis for professional confidentiality.

Confidentiality

According to Paul Finn (1992), in most professions, the notion of professional confidentiality implies four propositions:

1) information is not limited to that actually communicated by the client to the professional (it can include opinion derived from observation as well as the exercise of professional judgment);
2) the duration of the obligation extends beyond the period when a person has ceased to be a client;

3) the obligation can be overridden in some circumstances by other ethical considerations;

4) the obligation is subject to compliance with the law, at least when the specific law in question is ethically defensible.

These propositions help us understand the nature, and limits, of professional confidentiality. Importantly, proposition 3) means that the principle of confidentiality is not absolute. Under certain circumstances it can be overridden by other moral considerations, including ones which are enshrined in the law (as specified in proposition 4)). Such considerations include the rights of third parties at risk from clients. Here the legal requirement is fundamentally based on moral obligations. In this vein see case studies 8.1, 8.2, 8.3 and 8.6.

Moreover, confidentiality ought not be taken to be simply a matter of the right of a client. Proposition 1), for example, implies that confidentiality extends beyond what may transpire between client and social worker so that a social worker's opinions about a client may also need to be protected from disclosure. Additionally, propositions 3) and 4) seem to imply that the existence of confidential information concerning a client, whether known to that client or not, may not be subject to any control by that client.

At any rate when considering the principle of confidentiality in relation to information or opinion concerning a client, we need to ask whether it is

- client/practitioner confidentiality; or
- practitioner/practitioner confidentiality; or
- practitioner/employer confidentiality; or
- practitioner/third party confidentiality,

that is at issue. Our concern in the remainder of this chapter is with client/practitioner confidentiality, and confidentiality in respect of information or opinion concerning a client.

Since confidentiality is not an absolute principle, it may be overridden or restricted by other considerations. The question then is, on what basis should a decision be made when there is a clash between confidentiality and some other professional value. In many discussions of professional ethics confidentiality is treated as if it is, in itself, of great value. Any profession is, to some extent, free to choose which ethical rules and principles they wish to elevate or deem more important than others. It is nevertheless essential that these decisions are able to withstand rational scrutiny. Here we argue that in fact the value of confidentiality is derivative. Respecting confidentiality is valuable where it prevents harm, say, or facilitates the trust between professional and client that is necessary for effective practice. When this is acknowledged, many of the difficulties involving apparent conflicts between confidentiality and other values can be resolved.

Let us consider how confidentiality is necessary in certain settings to prevent harm. Think of police investigations into internal corruption or organised crime. If criminals come to know they are being investigated this may compromise the investigation. Indeed, if police are using undercover operatives or informants (see case study 8.5) then lives may be put at risk, if confidentiality is breached. So one important basis for professional confidentiality in certain settings is the likely serious harm, including loss of life, if confidentiality is not established and maintained.

Another argument commonly used to justify a very robust principle of confidentiality, especially in human service settings, is the so-called trust argument. Consider case study 8.3 (*Tarasoff v Regents of the University of California*, 1976). In their joint judgment the judges said that while there was a need to protect confidences generally it 'must yield to the extent to which disclosure is essential to avert danger to others. The protective privilege ends where the public peril begins ...'

The defence raised by the university was that the psychologist had an obligation to respect confidences arising in the course of a professional relationship. This obligation outweighed any other he might owe to the wider community, including Tatiana Tarasoff. The main argument offered in defence of the principle of confidentiality was an argument of trust. If confidentiality was violated, people would be deterred from seeking treatment, would be reluctant to fully disclose to their therapist, and the relationship between professional and client would be undermined because of a lack of trust. (See also case studies 8.2 and 8.4.)

Even if we acknowledge that confidentiality is necessary to preserve trust and thereby ensure the provision of psychological and other forms of treatment, it is highly implausible that the need for treatment overrides the rights to life of innocent third parties; especially when the lives in question are taken or threatened by those under treatment.

Let us now turn to the principle of confidentiality itself. What moral weight does it have, and what is the argument for giving it this weight?

The argument about loss of trust between client and professional underpins the elevation of the rule of confidentiality among many professionals – including doctors, journalists, social workers, psychologists – to the status of a basic and very robust principle. Trust is necessary for effective practice, and confidentiality is necessary for trust. Therefore confidentiality is a basic and very robust ethical principle in professional practice.

The force of this argument, as distinct from its validity, turns on the moral weight of effective practice. We will assume in what follows that effective work in the professions delivers human goods of very considerable moral weight, or at least does so in a significant number of cases.

While conceding that some extent of confidentiality is necessary for trust, and some extent of trust necessary for effective practice, it is by no means clear that a very robust principle of confidentiality is necessary for trust and hence for effective practice (Collingridge, Miller and Bowles 2001).

For one thing, scant conclusive empirical evidence for this claim exists. Marcia Neave, writing about HIV and confidentiality, observes that:

> Unfortunately there is little empirical evidence
> bearing upon this difficult policy question. The
> extent to which preservation of doctor–patient

> confidence affects willingness of individuals to
> seek medical help or to provide information about
> their sexual behaviour to their doctors is not really
> known ... Findings about ... the psychotherapists–
> patient/relationship (such as frankness of patients
> during interviews) have also been inconclusive
> (Neave 1987, p 4).

For another thing, the trust argument seems to have distorted the motivational relationship between confidentiality and effectiveness, at least from the client's perspective. A *reasonably high* level of confidentiality and trust is perhaps necessary for professional effectiveness. However, we also suggest that a low level of professional effectiveness can substantially contribute to the desire for a *very high* level of confidentiality. Sometimes, a client's concern that the professional may not be able to solve his problem will lead him to require airtight guarantees of confidentiality. Consider the high level of confidentiality demanded by HIV patients. On the other hand if the client knows the problem is going to be solved he is less concerned that its existence not be disclosed. If a cure for AIDS was discovered would not the demand for confidentiality weaken?

Another reason for the demand for a high level of confidentiality between workers and clients could be that it protects professionals from scrutiny of ineffective, or immoral practice. Consider the many cases of recent disclosure of sexual abuse between workers and clients during the course of therapy, or while the clients were in residential care.

If these lines of reasoning are sound, then the implication is that demands for robust confidentiality are likely to exist in professions in which there is often some doubt as to the effectiveness of their procedures or their practitioners.

So much for our characterisation of confidentiality as it is conceived in the professions and the importance attached to the trust argument. We have argued against placing great weight on the trust argument. We now claim that confidentiality is in some settings – but by no means all – derived from the notion of privacy.

Privacy

Let us first try to get clear on the notion of privacy. This is difficult to adequately explicate. However, a number of general points can be made (see generally, Benn 1988).

First, the notion of privacy has both a descriptive and a normative dimension. On the one hand, privacy consists of not being interfered with or having some power to exclude. On the other, privacy is held to be a moral right, or at least an important good. Most accounts of privacy acknowledge this much. For example, Warren and Brandeis (1890) gave an early and famous definition in terms of the 'right to be let alone'.

Naturally the normative and the descriptive dimensions interconnect. What ought to be, must be something that realistically could be. It is not realistic to think that the right to privacy could imply that other people should not look at you as you walk down the street. On the other hand, the mere fact that satellite cameras are now powerful enough to take images of residential backyards does not mean that the right to privacy cannot be invoked against corporations which wish to take and sell photos of people in their own homes.

Second, privacy is a desirable condition or power or a moral right that a person has in relation to other persons, and with respect to the acquisition of *information* by other persons about him/herself or the *observation/perceiving* of him/herself by other persons. The range of matters regarded as private embraces much of a person's *inner self*. A demand – as opposed to a request – by one person to know all about another person's thoughts, beliefs, emotions, and bodily sensations and states would be regarded as unacceptable. Some may thus deduce that privacy and secrecy are related concepts. Bok (1984) defines secrecy as intentional concealment whereas, according to Fried (1968), privacy is concerned with the control individuals have over information about themselves, as well as the ability to modulate the quality of the knowledge.

Third, privacy is a desirable condition or power or moral right that a person has in relation to other persons, with respect to the interference in the person's life by the other persons. (It is also taken to include protection from unwanted physical intrusions into one's private space.) In particular, a person's *intimate personal relations* with other people are regarded as private. So while a lover, friend or close relation might be entitled to know certain things or to intervene in a person's life, others would not be so entitled.

Fourth, certain facts are regarded as private by virtue of the impact of their disclosure on a person's various *public roles and practices* (Benn 1988). These kinds of facts are apparently regarded as private in part by virtue of the potential, should they be disclosed, of undermining the capacity of the person to function in these public roles or to fairly compete in these practices. If others know a person's criminal record, this may undermine their job prospects. If business competitors have access to my business plans, they will gain an unfair advantage over me. If a would-be employer knows my sexual preferences he or she may unfairly discriminate against me.

Fifth, Westin (1967) suggests that privacy is 'an instrument for achieving individual goals of self-realisation'. Thus, a measure of privacy is necessary simply so a person can pursue his or her projects, whatever those projects might be. For one thing reflection is necessary for planning, and this requires privacy. For another, knowledge of someone else's plans can enable those plans to be thwarted. *Autonomy* requires a measure of privacy. (See Chapter 7 for an account of autonomy.)

Given this account of privacy, what can we say of the relationship of privacy to confidentiality with special reference to human service professionals? At least two kinds of case exist in which confidentiality derives from the right to privacy.

First, there are circumstances under which a professional's knowledge concerning a client's inner self or intimate relations, are in the client's interest. A doctor needs to know about a patient's bodily sensations and states, in so far as this is necessary for successful treatment and in so far as the patient has consented to be treated; similarly for psychologists and social workers. This need to know for the benefit of the client gives rise to the principle of confidentiality. Such information, while available to the doctor or social worker, would still be unavailable to others, and for the doctor or social worker to disclose this information would constitute a breach of confidentiality.

Second, there are circumstances under which a social worker, or other professional, may legitimately interfere in the life of a client. This is notwithstanding that it is not in the client's interest, or at least notwithstanding the fact that the client has not given his or her informed consent. Such cases include ones in which the client is harming, or is likely to harm, some third party, and cases in which the client is harming or is likely to harm him/herself and is not able to give informed consent.

In these cases the professional has in fact infringed the privacy of the client, albeit possibly legitimately. It must be said that cases exist in which the right to privacy is invaded, and this tends to be glossed over. Human service professionals often have to involve themselves in the lives of others, and in doing so override their rights to privacy. In particular cases this may be justified. But it should not be assumed that there is a licence to do so, even when the outcome is likely to be good.

One of the implications of the right to privacy is that the invasion of privacy of a client, even if legitimate, needs to be contained. Thus, information gained in the course of such an invasion does not thereby automatically lose its status as private. This amounts to a requirement of confidentiality. But consider the problem which occurs in relation to familial genetic diseases where screening or testing reveals that other members of the family are carriers or recipients of the genetic disorder. In this sense, there may be no such thing as genetic privacy in a family context because the testing of one person must invade the privacy of another. It nevertheless raises troubling questions about the value of the professional/client confidential relationship.

Readings

Batty, David (2001) 'Calls to break addict confidentiality rejected', *The Guardian*, 7 March.

Benn, Stanley (1988) *A Theory of Freedom*, Cambridge University Press, Cambridge.

Bok, Sissela (1984) *Secrets: On the Ethics of Concealment and Revelation*, Oxford University Press, New York.

Collingridge, Michael, Miller, Seumas, and Bowles, Wendy (2001) 'Privacy and confidentiality in social work', *Australian Social Work*, vol 54(2), pp 3–14.

Finn, Paul (1992) 'Professionals and confidentiality', *Sydney Law Review*, vol 14, pp 317–39.

Fried, Charles (1968) 'Privacy', *Yale Law Journal*, vol 77, p 474.

Kuhse, Helga (1966) 'Confidentiality and the AMA's new code of ethics: An imprudent formulation?', *Medical Journal of Australia*, vol 165, pp 327–29.

Neave, Marcia (1987) 'Confidentiality and the duty to warn', *University of Tasmania Law Review*, vol 9, pp 1–31.

Office of Technology Assessment (1993) *Protecting Privacy in Computerised Medical Information*, US Government Printing Office, US Congress, Washington.

Rhodes, Margaret L (1986) *Ethical Dilemmas in Social Work Practice*, Routledge & Kegan Paul, Boston, p 56.

Tarasoff v Regents of the University of California (1976) 17 Cal 3d 358, Cal SC in Kuhse, Helga and Singer, Peter (eds) (1999) *Bioethics: An Anthology*, Blackwell, Oxford.

W v Edgell and Others (1990) 1 All ER 835 (QBD).

Warren, Samuel D and Brandeis, Louis D (1890) 'The right to privacy', *Harvard Law Review*, vol 4, no 1, p 4.

Westin, Alan F (1967) *Privacy and Freedom*, Atheneum, New York.

9: Life and death

When doctors warned [Miss B] in August 1999 that a malformation of blood vessels in her spinal column could result in severe disability, she wrote out a will expressly stating her wish not to receive treatment if she was left suffering from a life-threatening condition, permanent mental impairment or unconsciousness.

But when her condition improved, Miss B left hospital optimistic about her future and eventually returned to work.

However, at the beginning of 2001, she began to suffer weakening on the left side of her body and numbness in her legs. In February a massive recurrence of the bleeding left her tetraplegic, with complete paralysis from the neck down.

She was transferred to an intensive care unit, where she has been since, entirely dependent on a ventilator. At the time of her transfer she referred the two consultants treating her to her will, which stated that she did not want to be kept alive on a ventilator. But the doctors said her will was not specific enough to authorise them to end treatment.

After an operation that relieved her condition, allowing her to move her head and to speak, she again asked for the ventilator to be switched off.

156

By April, Miss B gave formal instructions via her solicitors for her treatment to cease and the hospital responded by calling in two independent psychiatrists to assess her competence to make the decision. Both initially found she did have such a capacity, but then reversed their findings.

While this was going on, preparations had been made for the ventilator to be switched off, and Miss B held discussions with one of the doctors, agreeing she should have three days to say goodbye to her friends and family and to finalise her affairs.

These preparations were called off when the psychiatrists changed their reports and Miss B was prescribed antidepressants. It was at this time that Miss B did agree she was relieved the ventilator had not been switched off and in May said she would try rehabilitation.

But in August Miss B authorised a doctor to reassess her ability to make decisions on her treatment and he found that she was competent. The hospital said it respected her decision, but did not turn off the ventilator.

Miss B today won her high court battle for the right to die. Dame Elizabeth Butler-Sloss, president of the high court family division, said the ruling would allow the woman to die 'peacefully and with dignity'. She can now effectively choose the time she wants to die; there has been no indication, however, when this might be.

[Miss B died on 24 April 2002.]

Mark Oliver (2002) 'The right-to-die judgment',
Guardian Unlimited, 22 March

CASE STUDY 9.2

I am only 43 years old. I desperately want a doctor to help me to die. Motor neurone disease has left my mind as sharp as ever, but it has gradually destroyed my muscles, making it hard for me to communicate with my family. It has left me in a wheelchair, catheterised and fed through a tube. I have fought against the disease for the last 2 years and had every possible medical treatment.

I am fully aware of what the future holds and have decided to refuse artificial ventilation. Rather than die by choking or suffocation, I want a doctor to help me die when I am no longer able to communicate with my family and friends. I have discussed this with my husband of 25 years, Brian who has come to terms with what I want and respects my decision. He says that losing me will be devastating for him and our two children but he would be pleased to know I had had the good death I want. I want to have a quick death without suffering, at home surrounded by my family so that I can say good-bye to them.

If I were physically able I could take my own life. That's not illegal. But because of the terrible nature of my illness I cannot take my own life – to carry out my wish I will need assistance. Should a doctor give me the assistance I need, he or she will be guilty of a crime that carries a lengthy prison sentence. As the law stands it makes no sense.

[Diane Pretty died on 11 May 2002, after losing her case in the European Court of Human Rights.]

Diane Pretty's account available at
<http://www.dignityindying.org.uk>

CASE STUDY 9.3

Many will remember the tragic case of Tony Bland, the 17-year-old football fan who was so badly injured in the Hillsborough football stadium disaster on 15 April 1989. Crushed up against the barriers, his brain was starved of oxygen. The severe and irreversible damage this caused meant that Mr Bland was diagnosed as being in a 'persistent vegetative state' (PVS). This condition has been described as 'awake but not aware'. Patients have no consciousness at all, but still retain the functions of breathing and circulation. They cannot see, hear, feel or think. Patients in PVS require intensive nursing care to survive, including the provision of artificial food and fluid.

Tony Bland's parents waited over three years before, coming to terms with the fact that their son was not going to recover, they decided to apply to the High Court to ask for treatment to be withdrawn, so he could die in peace. The law was unclear, and they did not wish to proceed until they had clear legal support. In November 1992, the Blands' case was successful in the High Court. Sir Stephen Brown, President of the Family Division, ruled that doctors may 'lawfully discontinue all life-sustaining treatment and medical support measures.'

Following an appeal from the Official Solicitor against this judgement, the case moved on to the Court of Appeal. By December, this court agreed that 'the withdrawal of medical care, including the removal of artificial feeding procedures, was not unlawful where the patient suffered from a persistent vegetative state from which he would not recover and where it was known that after such withdrawal, the patient would die.'

After the High Court and the Court of Appeals, finally it was the turn of the Law Lords to consider the case. Their verdict would be final. The Bland family had to wait until February 1993 before the unanimous ruling came – that artificial feeding should be withdrawn from their son. The ruling was backed by the British Medical Association.

After this long process of court decision and appeal, treatment was finally withdrawn from Tony Bland. He died on 3 March 1993, with his parents by his side.

Jenni Burt's account is available at
<http://www.dignityindying.org.uk>

CASE STUDY 9.4

In July 1949 Leo Alexander, Chief US Medical Consultant at the Nuremberg Crimes Trials, published his essay 'Medical Science Under Dictatorship.' It is still considered a classic piece of research. The Nazi rule in Germany was preceded by 'a propaganda barrage directed against the traditional compassionate nineteenth-century attitudes towards the chronically ill', Alexander writes. 'Sterilization and euthanasia of persons with chronic illnesses was discussed at a meeting of Bavarian psychiatrists in 1931.' Alexander's main concern was the shift in medical ethics and attitudes after January 1933 when Hitler was appointed Reichchancellor: 'Nazi propaganda was highly effective in perverting public opinion and public conscience in a remarkably short time. In the medical profession this expressed itself in a rapid decline in standards of professional ethics.'

The crimes which the Nazis would commit later had their origins in prior subtle changes as stated in the following:

> The beginnings at first were merely a subtle shift in emphasis in the basic attitude of the physicians. It started with the acceptance of the attitude, basic in the euthanasia movement, that there is such a thing as life not worthy to be lived. This attitude in its early stages concerned itself merely with the severely and chronically sick. Gradually the sphere of those to be included in this category was enlarged to encompass the socially unproductive, the ideologically unwanted, the racially unwanted and finally all non-Germans.

At medical facilities the principle that physicians must fight for the life of their patients in accordance with the Hippocratic Oath came under attack. In Alexander's view this did not happen overnight, it happened gradually … Alexander points out that 'by 1936 extermination of the physically or socially unfit was so openly accepted that its practice was mentioned incidentally in an article in an official German medical journal.' …

Alexander's observations about 'small beginnings' and 'subtle shift' refer to an 'early change in medical attitudes' and 'a propaganda barrage even before the Nazis took open charge.' The notion 'that there is such a thing as life not worthy to be lived' marked the starting point. This was before the Nazis came to power. Alexander fully recognizes that the year 1933 was crucial as he mentions the effectiveness of Nazi propaganda early on. The coming to power of the Nazis in 1933 accelerated things and culminated six years later in Hitler's Euthanasia Decree which was deliberately couched in cautious language (in practice it gave a free rein to those who practiced mass killings).

John Arthur Emerson Vermaat (2002) 'Euthanasia in the Third Reich: Lessons for today?' *Ethics & Medicine*

In her late sixties Australian Nancy Crick had a series of operations for bowel cancer. Despite the operations she continued to suffer from ongoing debilitating pain. In February, 2002, Crick gave a press conference at which she indicated that she was going to take her own life before the winter, and was going to establish a website diary to record her thoughts and progress during the last few months of her life. While the diary bore Crick's name, it was, in fact, a group effort. Australia's 'Dr Death', Dr Philip Nitschke, and his newly formed pro-euthanasia organization, Exit Australia, provided the computer and the web site software, as well as 'Internet helpers' to actually post the diary entries. Nitschke was particularly helpful and supportive, Crick said, as was John Edge, also from Exit Australia, who served as her media front man and secretary. She was also receiving assistance from the Voluntary Euthanasia Society of Queensland. As well as helping with her web diary, members of Exit Australia organised an effective media campaign publicising Crick's situation.

Throughout the diary, Crick described her diminished life with bowel cancer. 'I have bowel cancer and it is bloody painful ... I was recently asked how much had my life style changed since the discovery of bowel cancer', she wrote. 'Things changed dramatically after the first bowel operation', she explained, 'no more window shopping, no swimming with my mates, no bingo, no longer free and easy, [sic] I became ever increasingly bonded to my toilet in a "Till death do us part" relationship.'

The fear of being dependent and a burden was Crick's underlying motivation for death. Crick's son, Wayne Crick, told reporters after her death that his mother had told him and his younger brother, Daryle, that she was determined to end her life to stop her suffering and to make sure that she did not become a burden on her family.

Concerned that his mother was being used by the euthanasia movement, Wayne recounted, 'I said to her one day: "Mum, they are using you", and she said: "Yes, I know, but I'm using them."'

On May 22nd, with 21 friends and family present, Crick took a lethal dose of barbiturates with a draught of 'Bailey's', and after a few puffs on a last cigarette, went quickly to sleep and died within 20 minutes.

According to the Brisbane pathologist who performed Crick's autopsy, she did not have cancer when she died. There was evidence that she had cancer prior to her first surgery several years ago, but he could find no visual trace of the cancer anywhere in her body now. What she did have was a 'twisted bowel' and some minor illnesses which caused her discomfort.

Euthanasia advocates shifted quickly into damage control mode. 'All the evidence points to the fact that she died because she considered herself terminally ill and that's the end of the story', said Exit Australia's John Edge.

A second shock wave soon followed: both Crick and Dr Nitschke knew she was cancer-free, and told no-one – not even her immediate family! Two months prior to Crick's death, Gold Coast Hospital's palliative care director, Dr Barbara Craig, met with both Crick and Nitschke and informed them that Crick did not have cancer. Other claims made over the course of Crick's campaign were also found to be false. Crick was not dying of malnutrition, and she was not 27 kg (60 lbs) as she stated in her diary and as Nitschke told the press. Medical records showed her weight as 36 kg (79 lbs) in 2001 and 38 kg (84 lbs) just weeks before she died.

Melbourne University professor of palliative care Dr David Kissane called the euthanasia campaign an example of the slippery slope phenomenon where right-to-diers say 'terminally ill', but mean 'hopelessly ill'. 'The euthanasia movement denies the slippery slope argument, they say it won't happen. But we've just seen, in real time, precisely that happen with Nancy Crick', he said.

Adapted from International Task Force on Euthanasia and Assisted Suicide (2002) *Special Report: The Death that Backfired on the Right-to-Die Movement*

ETHICAL ANALYSIS

Death

The will to live is a fundamental drive in all sentient beings. Correspondingly, death is generally seen as a great evil to be avoided, if possible. Our social arrangements reflect these deep-seated attitudes to life and death. We invest huge sums of money in medical technology, public health measures and safety devices to extend life and ward off death. Murder, the intentional taking of another's life, is punished with great severity.

Obviously, most of the time, most of us want to go on living. However, some of the time, some of us don't. In Australia, suicide ranks as one of the major killers of young people: a quarter of the deaths of males aged between 15 and 24 are suicides, for example.

Much more effective and widely available medical treatments have meant that our lives can be protracted far longer than was previously possible. While overall this is obviously a great boon, it has also created situations where continued prolongation of life actually appears undesirable (see case studies 9.1 and 9.3). This has stimulated discussion of the moral permissibility of withdrawal of life-preserving medical treatment, medically assisted suicide (where a doctor provides a patient with the means to kill themselves) and euthanasia (where a doctor kills a patient for compassionate reasons).

Given the great value we place on the preservation of life, it is not surprising that claims that people have a right to end their own lives, help others in doing so, or even in some cases end the lives of other people, are controversial. In examining such claims we need to address two sets of questions. The first concerns the moral status of acts such as suicide and euthanasia. The second asks what public policy should be in regard to such acts: what kinds of laws, institutional arrangements and so on should we have in these cases? The moral status of actions is obviously relevant to decisions we make about public policy: other things being equal, it is desirable to have policy that encourages or mandates morally good actions, and that discourages or even prevents morally bad actions. However, things are not always equal. Sometimes, for example, the only effective means to prevent morally bad kinds of actions is so costly, intrusive, or otherwise undesirable that it is preferable not to avail ourselves of it. Sometimes policy that aims to encourage morally good outcomes has such terrible unintended side-effects that it does more harm than good.

A right to die?

Most people agree that there is a moral right to life, and that given such a right it is morally wrong to kill people. Naturally, in some circumstances, such as self-defence, a person's right to life (for example, the right to life of an attacker) can be overridden. However, the right to life can be overridden only by very weighty moral considerations and in highly restricted circumstances. Thus a person is morally justified in killing an attacker in self-defence, but only if it is necessary in order to preserve their life.

Moreover, the concept of human life in play here is itself problematic. Ordinarily being alive consists in having consciousness, being able to think, form intentions, imagine possibilities, perform actions, perceive the physical world, communicate with other human beings, experience sensations of pain and pleasure, and so on. However, on medical definitions of human life, a person is only dead if they are brain dead or if they have ceased to breathe. (See case study 9.3.)

Notwithstanding problems with the definition of human life we can distinguish between being alive and the quality of that life. For example, someone in prison is clearly alive, but suffering a diminution in their autonomy, and someone with AIDS is alive, but suffering poor health and (in all probability) considerable pain. Being alive is generally regarded as a good in itself, as well as a necessary condition for other goods, such as autonomy. However, there are circumstances in which we would be better off dead: consider a person who is being slowly tortured to death.

A focus on persons who are experiencing extreme suffering with no prospect of relief, and/or are physically incapacitated and terminally ill, and/or are barely alive by virtue of having lost such central mental faculties as the ability to think or be conscious, has led many to think that suicide, euthanasia and the like might be morally justifiable. Those who think this, often appeal to the existence of a supposed 'right to die'. This (alleged) right implies (at least) that individuals are entitled to decide for themselves the manner and time at which they die.

It is controversial whether or not there is a basic right to die, as opposed to a non-absolute right to life that can be overridden in certain highly restricted circumstances. However, it is now generally accepted that people ought to be allowed to refuse medical treatment, even if the consequence of such refusal will be that they die; where, as we say, we let 'nature take its course'. What is more controversial is whether it is morally permissible to choose to act in a way that brings about death when it would not otherwise have occurred, for instance in suicide or euthanasia.

The concept of a moral right is a complex one. However, in the case of at least some moral rights, including the right to die (assuming it exists) possession of the right implies that others should not prevent the holder of the right from exercising it (Thomson 1990). Thus, if someone has a moral right to kill themselves, and they choose to do so, then others should not intervene to preserve their life. On the other hand, another person is entitled to intervene to try to convince the person not to choose to exercise their right by, say, trying to talk them out of committing suicide.

From the fact that someone has a moral right and chooses to exercise it, it does not follow that they are doing what is best or even acting in a morally good way. If someone has a property right over a valuable painting, for example, they are entitled to destroy the painting, even though that would be a bad thing to do. The question of whether we should accept that there is a moral right to act in a certain way, then, is logically prior to the question of how we should judge the action of someone who acts in accordance with their right.

Arguments for the existence of a right to die appeal either to autonomy, or to compassion, or to both (Rachels 1986). Autonomy is a fundamental moral value. Moreover, there is a strong presumption in favour of respecting a person's autonomy when that person is not harming anyone else. Accordingly, we think twice about infringing a person's autonomy when they are only harming themself, by marrying a bad person, say, or giving up their well-paid job to become a beach-bum. On the other hand, if someone was to autonomously choose to give up their autonomy, by choosing to become a slave, say, then we might regard this as morally unacceptable, and seek to prevent it. At the very least it seems paradoxical to exhibit one's respect for another's autonomy by allowing them to extinguish it. Likewise, we might value human life to the point that we believe it to be morally unacceptable to allow someone to autonomously choose to kill themselves. Whether or not we should intervene might depend, in part, on whether we value autonomy above life. If we value someone's autonomy above their life, then perhaps we should allow them to autonomously kill themself. However, matters are not quite so simple. For in allowing them to kill themselves we are allowing them to extinguish their autonomy; if no life, then no autonomy.

The second consideration commonly appealed to ground the right to die is that of compassion. It is claimed that just as compassion – being moved by others' suffering – often provides grounds for helping people to continue their lives, on occasions the compassionate thing to do is to allow, or even assist, others to die. Without life, we cannot experience any goods. Hence, when helping someone to stay alive (by providing food to the survivors of a natural disaster, for example) will enable them to go on to live a worthwhile life, compassion counsels us to do so. In some cases, however, continued life brings with it burdens (or costs), such as severe physical and mental pain and a diminution in autonomy, that far outweigh the benefits from being alive. Surely, at some point the burdens are so great and the benefits so limited that one's life is simply not worth living, as in the case mentioned above of the person being tortured to death. In such circumstances, it would seem that compassion would counsel us to allow someone to take their own life, at least, and perhaps even to help them do so. While this argument might be compelling – depending on what the benefits and burdens on the ledger are – it does not demonstrate that there is a moral right to die. It merely posits that the right to, or value of, life can be overridden in certain restricted circumstances, namely extreme suffering and a diminution in autonomy.

The above argument, while it appeals to compassion, also invites us to weigh the costs and benefits associated with two incompatible courses of action, namely, the act of terminating a life as opposed to refraining from ending that life. However, this kind of moral cost/benefit analysis is resisted by some moral theorists, notably, by Immanuel Kant and his followers.

Kant enunciated a deep intuition about the appropriate way of dealing with autonomous beings, famously telling us to 'Act so that you treat humanity, whether in your own person or in that of another, always as an end and never as a means only' (Kant 1998). Acts such as theft and assault are wrong not simply because they harm their victims, but because they disrespect them, in the sense that the wrongdoer acts as if the victim is simply an inanimate thing without intentions and ends of its own. So we are likely to be upset by being robbed, even if we disliked the things taken and wanted to get rid of them. For Kant, we can exhibit disrespect in this sense even when we are motivated by altruistic, rather than selfish, considerations. Consider a society in which when someone turns 25 a decision is made as to whether they are allowed to go on living or will be executed. This decision is based on an informed judgment as to whether, all things considered, their continued existence is likely to be a benefit or a burden to the society. While such cost/benefit calculations are suitable when we are faced with economic decisions such as whether to keep a power plant operational, they are surely unacceptable as a guide to the appropriate way to treat people. They are, as we say, inhuman. From the Kantian point of view they overlook the fact that individual lives have value in themselves, irrespective of the consequences of the way those lives are lived. Moreover, as we saw in Chapter 3, the value of one human life is not commensurable, numerically speaking, with the value of a second human life. But if it is wrong for someone to use cost/benefit calculations to decide whether others should live or die, surely it is wrong for them to use such calculations to decide whether they themselves should live or die, choosing to die, say, when they judge that the burdens of continued existence will outweigh any possible benefits.

Even if we accept the Kantian objection to moral cost/benefit analysis, there is surely an argument to be made in favour of terminating a life. Here we need to distinguish two situations. In the first, if we do not end our own life, we will go on living for an indefinite time. In the second situation, we are definitely going to die, as we are suffering from a terminal illness. In the latter case, we cannot decide whether we will die: that is a given. We can, however, still decide how we will die. In such cases, is it really disrespectful of our status as autonomous beings who are valuable in ourselves to wish to die a painless death, with our faculties intact? (Consider here Diane Pretty's situation, described in case study 9.2.)

A right to kill?

If we accept that there is a right to die, what follows? At least, the right to die seems to entail that there is a right to take one's own life (even if only in special circumstances). If we are permitted to take our own life, does this mean that others are permitted to help us take it? The existence of a right to die is one way to justify the moral permissibility of taking my own life. However, if I am not permitted to take my own life, then presumably others cannot be justified in helping me to do so. And even if we do have a right to take our own life, others might not be justified in helping us. In general, from the fact that one person has a right to act in a certain way, it does not automatically follow that others are entitled to help them. A liberal approach to morality, for example, advocates that people have a right to act as they want in respect of self-regarding actions, that is, actions that do not harm others. So a person with no dependants may have a right to drink themselves to death. Surely it does not follow that someone who helps them achieve this end by, say, buying alcohol for them when they are too hung-over to do so themselves, or giving them money to buy drink, is acting in a morally acceptable way.

Similarly, even if we accept that people have a right to take their own life, it does not automatically follow that there can be no objection to others helping them, by providing the means for them to do so (in assisted suicide) or doing it for them if they are unwilling or unable to do so themselves (in euthanasia). Rather we will have to consider the moral status of such assistance on a case by case basis. Sometimes, where for example a person is facing a painful and protracted terminal illness (as in the case of Diane Pretty, discussed in case study 9.2), assisting others to die may be morally permissible, or even good, while in others, for example where a healthy young person is temporarily depressed over a failed romance, or where a sick person has been persuaded by grasping relatives that her going on living would be selfish, it should be condemned.

Euthanasia: morality

The word 'euthanasia' derives from two Greek words, '*eu*' (good), and '*thanatos*' (death). Accordingly, euthanasia involves the intentional ending of the life of a person in order to relieve their suffering, or otherwise for their own good.

Since most of the recent controversy focusses on euthanasia in hospital settings, where the stricken person is a patient and the person who is faced with a choice about how to treat them is a doctor, we will assume that setting in the following discussion. There are a number of things to note about euthanasia. Firstly, it only occurs when a person's life has been intentionally ended. So killing a patient will not count as euthanasia if it is accidental; nor if the killing is a foreseen but not intended consequence of something done. A doctor, for example, may hasten death by prescribing a heavy dose of pain-killing drugs. If their intention is to ease the patient's pain, not to kill them, this will not count as euthanasia. Secondly, euthanasia can only occur when the intentional ending of a life is motivated by the desire to relieve the suffering of the person whose life is ended. If it is otherwise motivated, it may well be murder, even if it results in the relief of suffering. Indeed, some cases of euthanasia may, nevertheless, be cases of wrongful killing (depending on one's moral beliefs about the cases of euthanasia in question).

There are a number of different kinds of euthanasia. Firstly, there is passive euthanasia, where a patient is allowed to die by withdrawing treatment, life support (respirator etc), or ongoing intervention. Secondly, there is active euthanasia, where a patient is killed through, for example, the administration of a lethal dose of drugs. Whether active or passive, we can further distinguish acts of euthanasia according to whether they are voluntary (where the patient expresses rational, considered desire to be euthanased, as in case study 9.2), non-voluntary (where the patient has not expressed a rational, considered wish about euthanasia, as in case study 9.3), or involuntary (where a patient has expressed a rational, considered desire not to be euthanased).

As we noted above, the claim that voluntary passive euthanasia is morally *permissible* under certain circumstances is widely accepted in the Australian community. We have a right to refuse medical treatment if we so desire. Similarly, the claim that involuntary (passive or active) euthanasia is morally *impermissible* is generally accepted. That is, we ought not kill people who do not wish to die, even if they are suffering from a terminal illness, nor should we withdraw effective treatment against the wishes of the ill. There remains a good deal of controversy about the status of non-voluntary passive euthanasia. Recent public opinion and legal judgment has tended to agree that such euthanasia can be justified in the case of terminally ill patients existing under certain conditions of infirmity and/or suffering and where continued medical treatment would be burdensome or futile. (See case study 9.3.) On the other hand, the status of active euthanasia, even when it is voluntary, remains highly contested (see case study 9.1), and it remains illegal almost everywhere.

A vast philosophical literature now presents arguments for and against the moral permissibility of active euthanasia. Here we look at arguments based on the role morality of doctors.

As we saw in Chapter 6, the assumption of a professional role brings with it role-specific rights and duties, the content of which are determined by the defining end of the role. This fact about the nature of professional morality has been used to argue both against, and in favour of, the permissibility of euthanasia. Opponents of euthanasia have claimed that the end or purpose which defines the doctor's role is the preservation and restoration of healthy human functioning. Killing involves the ending of human functioning, so it is directly contradictory to doctors' defining end. And since active euthanasia is a form of killing, they have a duty, as doctors, not to engage in it, even in situations where there might be other reasons to do so. (Case study 9.4 illustrates what can happen when doctors lose sight of this duty.)

Some claim that such a definition of the doctor's role is too narrow. The ultimate goal of doctors is to use their medical skill to help their patients. However, this seems to accord too wide a professional role to doctors. We suggest that the role of a doctor is to preserve life and health, but to do so within certain limits. Specifically, it is not part of a doctor's role to preserve life come what may and, therefore, not part of a doctor's role to keep a terminally ill patient alive when they are suffering extreme pain, diminished autonomy, and there is no possibility of reducing their pain or enhancing their autonomy. Accordingly, in such circumstances a doctor ought to recommend against the continuation of futile or excessively burdensome treatment. It is no doubt that this kind of reasoning has brought about the wide acceptance of passive euthanasia, among the general public and the medical profession.

The same reasoning which has been used to support passive euthanasia in these sorts of cases, is also appealed to in support of active euthanasia. Consider the Diane Pretty case (case study 9.2). Past a certain point, medical treatment was useless in protracting Diane Pretty's life. At that point, her doctor had at least two reasons to discontinue treatment. The first involved an appeal to compassion: continued treatment would not be helpful, and may be burdensome. Therefore Diane would be better off without it. This gives a reason for a doctor motivated by concern for her welfare to stop treatment. The second reason was respect for autonomy: Diane had made a considered judgment against continued treatment (this is implicit in her wish to have help in dying). The same considerations speak in favour of her doctor not simply withdrawing treatment, but taking active steps to end her life. It is clear that merely withdrawing treatment will lead to Diane dying a slow and agonising death through choking and suffocation. How could someone motivated by compassion stand by and watch this happen when they have the capacity to bring about a quick and painless death? (Think of what we do when we kill suffering animals 'humanely'.) Secondly, Diane has expressed an explicit, considered and well-informed request for medical help in bringing her life to an end. We have no reason to think that this was not a fully autonomous request. In acting in accordance with it, a doctor therefore would be showing respect for Diane's autonomy.

There seem to be reasons, then, to hold that if we accept that passive euthanasia can be justified given certain conditions, we should also accept that active euthanasia can be justified when those same conditions hold. This conclusion, however, is often resisted by appealing to the supposed moral difference between letting die (a species of allowing), and killing (a species of doing). It is claimed while letting die is not itself necessarily a bad thing, killing is. Since passive euthanasia involves letting someone die, while active euthanasia involves killing them, there is a morally significant difference between an act of passive and active euthanasia, even if all the circumstances are the same. Hence, the argument goes, even if we accept that passive euthanasia is justified, we are not forced to agree that active euthanasia is as well.

One response to this claim has been to deny that there is any intrinsic difference between killing and letting die (Rachels 1986). No doubt, usually killing is (very) bad, and worse than letting die, because it is driven by hatred or some other vicious motivation, requires effort, is against the wishes of the person killed, and so on. But these are facts about the typical setting of killing, not essential features of killing itself. In some unusual cases, none of the facts that typically make killing wrong hold. In those cases, not only may killing not be bad, it may actually be good.

The question of whether killing is bad in itself remains contested. If we accept that it is, in contradiction to the argument just considered, then active euthanasia is, in itself a bad thing, since it involves killing. This does not, however, demonstrate that it is wrong. After all, many of the things that doctors do in the course of their medical activities are bad in themselves. Think, for example, of a doctor amputating a patient's gangrenous leg. Amputating a limb certainly looks like something that is bad in itself. To call an action bad (in itself) does not show that it cannot be justified; it does show that it requires justification. In the case of the gangrenous leg the justification is straightforward: the amputation is a necessary evil to prevent the far greater evil of death. In effect, the doctor is faced with a choice between two actions that will lead to two pairs of associated possible outcomes. If she chooses not to amputate, the outcome will be the preservation of the whole limb, together with the death of the patient. On the other hand, if she chooses to amputate, the outcome will be the loss of the limb, together with the continued life of the patient. The doctor is justified (in fact required) to choose the second pairing of action and outcome, and so is justified in amputating the leg as a necessary means to saving the patient's life, even though she would not have been justified in amputating it if were not a necessary means to achieve that goal. (This argument assumes that the patient has consented and that survival without one's limb is a far greater good than death with one's limb intact.) Note that this argument does not demonstrate that there is no moral difference between doing and allowing, but merely that in the kinds of example in question this makes no difference given the weight of the other moral considerations in play.

We can find a similar pattern of justification for certain cases of euthanasia. As claimed above, though generally life is a good, sometimes it can be a burden; some lives are not worth living (and are experienced as such). Consider a situation where a patient with a terminal illness is suffering intense pain which cannot be relieved. The patient's doctor, however, can end the suffering by administering a dose of a fatal drug. In such a situation, the patient's doctor is again faced with a choice between two courses of action, which will lead to two pairs of outcomes. She can decide not to administer the drugs, which have the effect of preserving the patient's life for a relatively brief period, and perpetuating their suffering. Or she can decide to administer the drugs, which will terminate the patient's life and end their suffering. Let us accept that the evil consequent on reducing the period of this terminally ill patient's life by providing them with a lethal drug is much less weighty than the suffering they would undergo if that drug is not administered. That is, we accept that the patient's life has become not worth living. The doctor thus seems to be justified in choosing to administer the fatal dose of drugs, with the intention of bringing about the patient's death, as a means to ending their suffering (and assuming that the patient has consented to this). That is, the doctor is morally justified in engaging in active euthanasia.

Euthanasia: legal policy

Much of the on-going debate over euthanasia has focussed on the legal status of physician-assisted suicide and voluntary active euthanasia. Polls in countries such as Australia indicate strong (over 80 percent) and persisting community support for legalising these activities. At the same time, they face deeply entrenched opposition and they remain illegal almost everywhere (with the exceptions of Netherlands, Belgium and the US state of Oregon). In a democratic society the existence of a clear and persistent majority preference for a change in the law provides a strong, if not decisive, reason in favour of such a change. Of course, the mere fact that a majority of people favours some course of action does not make it morally right or even pragmatically advisable. (Think, for example, of the 'White Australia' policy, which prevented non-European migration to Australia, and had broad support well into the 20th century.) However, even if we accept that euthanasia is (very) morally bad, this is not sufficient to show that it should remain illegal. We have good reason to believe that euthanasia will occur whether or not it is illegal. We also have reason to believe that when it is illegal, it is easy to conceal and even abuse. This provides another reason to legalise voluntary euthanasia, since legal euthanasia can be monitored and controlled. (This kind of reasoning has been influential in the legalisation of prostitution, and 'harm minimisation' programs aimed at drug users, for example.)

These are considerations in favour of legalising euthanasia that should weigh even for those who consider euthanasia to be morally bad. However, there are also considerations against legalisation, which also should weigh even for those who think that euthanasia can be morally justified in particular cases. The legalisation of voluntary euthanasia commits us to the adoption of a social policy. This means that we commit ourselves to acting – or allowing others to act – in a certain way whenever certain conditions apply.

Often, the adoption of a social policy is justified on consequentialist grounds. We are better off, for a range of reasons, in deciding on a rule for the allocation of a good (or burden) whenever we face a certain kind of situation, rather than having to work out how to act each time we face that kind of situation. A government, for example, may wish to provide financial support to academically capable people to attend university. These people would otherwise be excluded by lack of financial resources. It is decided to do this by instituting a policy of giving student grants to applicants who have finished high school and whose parents have an income of less than $30 000 per annum. Instituting this policy has at least two advantages over judging on a case-by-case basis. Firstly, it is much cheaper and easier to administer. Secondly, it removes the need for the exercise of discretionary judgment on the part of officials, thus making it less likely that personal biases and idiosyncrasies will infect the decision-making process, with similarly placed applicants being treated differently.

There are two ways in which policies of this kind can go wrong. Firstly, where those who should be designated as eligible for a service or good are passed over (we call this a Type One mistake); and secondly, where those who should not be so designated are nevertheless so designated (we call this a Type Two mistake). In the case of our student grant example, a Type One mistake occurs when an academically capable person who will be unable to attend university because of lack of financial resources is denied a grant. A Type Two mistake occurs when someone who already has sufficient financial resources is nevertheless given a grant. Many (maybe even all) social policies will produce both Type One and Type Two mistakes. We can make Type Two mistakes less likely, by tightening and enforcing the conditions of eligibility. The cost of doing so is that we make Type One mistakes more likely. On the other hand, we can make Type One mistakes less likely by loosening the conditions of eligibility – at the cost of increasing Type Two mistakes. In many cases, we are satisfied with a policy which steers a kind of middle road: not so stringent as to generate unacceptably large numbers of Type One mistakes, nor so loose as to produce too many Type Two mistakes. Policies of the kind we are considering may be justified if they do a good enough job, by and large and on the whole. As it is often put, social policy is a 'blunt instrument'. So our grant policy may be considered to be working if it is generally facilitating access to university education to those who would otherwise be excluded because of financial disadvantage. This would apply even if in some cases grants are given to the undeserving, or denied to those who need them.

Now let us apply this discussion to voluntary active euthanasia. Those who support relaxing the current legal prohibition think that there are good moral reasons to allow doctors to carry out euthanasia at least when certain conditions are met. These are that the person to be euthanased is competent to make a rational choice, and has expressed a freely chosen, considered and settled wish to have their life ended, and has done so for good reasons (in particular because they wish to relieve their suffering). They further believe that it is possible to institute a policy which will allow euthanasia in, and only in, such circumstances. Typically they will recommend, for example, that such a policy will require that a person can only be euthanased when they have signed a form requesting it, have been given counselling and time to change their mind, have been certified by a qualified person as mentally competent and not suffering from depression, and so on.

Again, there are two types of mistakes which could be made in the application of such a policy. A Type One mistake occurs when euthanasia is denied to a person who wants it, and where it would be morally justified. A Type Two mistake occurs when someone is euthanased though euthanasia is not morally justified. A Type Two mistake could occur, for example, when someone whose rationality is impaired by depression (and so is less than fully competent) asks to be euthanased, or when a competent person makes such a request because they feel have become a burden to others. (Consider the Nancy Crick case discussed in case study 9.5: what considerations may have influenced her?)

Making a Type Two mistake in the application of a policy of euthanasia would obviously be highly problematic. It would mean intentionally bringing about the death of a person who ought not to have been killed. Of course, the problems associated with Type Two mistakes only count against a policy that permits euthanasia if there is a realistic likelihood that such mistakes would be made. But we do have good reason to believe that such mistakes will be made, based on our experience of capital punishment. We now know that a number of innocent people have been executed in jurisdictions that permit capital punishment, despite the executions occurring after a rigorous trial process. If mistakes of this type seem to be an unavoidable consequence of a policy of allowing capital punishment given the satisfaction of certain procedural requirements, it seems highly probable that they would also occur if we introduced a policy of allowing euthanasia provided procedural requirements were satisfied.

Killing people who should not be killed is such a great wrong that it provides an extremely weighty reason against instituting a policy that will make it likely that this will occur. The most obvious way of avoiding Type Two mistakes is to prevent euthanasia; to retain and vigorously enforce its legal prohibition. On the other hand, the more restrictive our policy in relation to euthanasia, as we make it more likely that we will avoid Type Two mistakes, we make it more likely that we will commit Type One mistakes: those we think have a moral claim to have access to euthanasia are denied that access. The certainty that an effective policy of prohibition will generate Type One mistakes is, again, a weighty consideration against a policy of that kind.

One response to this dilemma is to adopt a kind of 'middle of road' policy that allows a certain number of both types of mistakes, so that we accept that some people who should not be euthanased will be, and that some who should have access to euthanasia will not. After all, this kind of approach seemed reasonable in the case of student grants. However, arguably this kind of approach will not do here. Intentionally killing those who should not be killed involves inflicting a very great and irreversible wrong on them. This is the primary reason to avoid allowing it to happen if at all possible. Moreover, it also involves those who carry out the killing (and less directly those who authorise it) in the commission of that very great wrong. Though not allowing those who have a moral claim to euthanasia to have access to it also involves considerable moral costs, these do not seem to have the same weight. The suffering of the terminally ill, for example, is by definition finite, and can often be mitigated. And while knowing that we could have helped relieve someone's suffering, but did not, may be morally painful, it is presumably not as morally damaging as fearing, or discovering, that we have killed someone who should not have been killed.

Finally, we should reiterate that our discussion in this section has focussed on legal policy, which is concerned with actions and choices in as much as they belong to certain general categories. It is worth recalling that even where there are overwhelmingly good reasons to adopt laws forbidding certain kinds of action, there may still be particular cases where an action of that kind is morally correct.

Readings

Dignity in Dying <http://www.dignityindying.org.uk> (accessed 23/1/09).

Glover, Jonathan (1977) *Causing Death and Saving Lives*, Penguin, Harmondsworth.

International Task Force on Euthanasia and Assisted Suicide (2002) *Special Report: The Death that Backfired on the Right-to-Die Movement*, vol 16, no 2, available at <http://www.internationaltaskforce.org/iua25.htm 2> (accessed 23/1/09).

Jarvis Thomson, Judith (1990) *Realm of Rights*, Harvard University Press, Cambridge.

Kant, Immanuel (1785, 1998) *Groundwork of the Metaphysic of Morals*, Gregor, Mary (editor and translator), with an introduction by Korsgaard, Christine, Cambridge University Press, Cambridge.

McMahan, Jeff (2002) *The Ethics of Killing: Problems at the Margins of Life*, Oxford University Press, New York.

Norcross, Alastair and Steinbock, Bonnie (1994) *Killing and Letting Die*, 2nd edition, Fordham University Press, New York.

Oliver, Mark (2002) 'The right-to-die judgment', *Guardian Unlimited*, 22 March, available at <http://www.guardian.co.uk> (accessed 23/1/09).

Rachels, James (1986) *The End of Life: Euthanasia and Morality*, Oxford University Press, Oxford.

Rosenbaum, Stuart and Baird, Robert (eds) (1989) *Euthanasia: The Moral Issues* Prometheus Books, Buffalo.

Tooley, Michael (1985) *Abortion and Infanticide*, Oxford University Press, Oxford.

Vermaat, John Arthur Emerson (2002) 'Euthanasia in the Third Reich: Lessons for today?', *Ethics & Medicine*, vol 18, p 1.

10: Reproduction

[The 'eugenics' movement – aiming to improve the quality of the human race through selective breeding – arose in Victorian England. It was embraced by politically influential groups in early 20th century America, alarmed by the rapid population growth of 'inferior' racial and class groups.]

[T]he main solution for eugenicists was the rapid expansion of forced segregation and sterilization, as well as more marriage restrictions. California led the nation, performing nearly all sterilization procedures with little or no due process. In its first twenty-five years of eugenic legislation, California sterilized 9782 individuals, mostly women. Many were classified as 'bad girls', diagnosed as 'passionate', 'oversexed' or 'sexually wayward.' At Sonoma, some women were sterilized because of what was deemed an abnormally large clitoris or labia.

In 1933 alone, at least 1278 coercive sterilizations were performed, 700 of which were on women. The state's two leading sterilization mills in 1933 were Sonoma State Home with 388 operations and Patton State Hospital with 363 operations. Other sterilization centers included Agnews, Mendocino, Napa, Norwalk, Stockton and

Pacific Colony state hospitals.

Even the United States Supreme Court endorsed aspects of eugenics. In its infamous 1927 decision, Supreme Court Justice Oliver Wendell Holmes wrote, 'It is better for all the world, if instead of waiting to execute degenerate offspring for crime, or to let them starve for their imbecility, society can prevent those who are manifestly unfit from continuing their kind ... Three generations of imbeciles are enough.' This decision opened the floodgates for thousands to be coercively sterilized or otherwise persecuted as subhuman ...

Only after eugenics became entrenched in the United States was the campaign transplanted into Germany, in no small measure through the efforts of California eugenicists, who published booklets idealizing sterilization and circulated them to German official[s] and scientists.

Edwin Black (2003) 'The horrifying American roots of Nazi eugenics', *History News Network*, 24 November

CASE STUDY 10.2

'Bokanovsky's Process', repeated the Director, and the students underlined the words in their little note-books.

One egg, one embryo, one adult – normality. But a bokanovskified egg will bud, will proliferate, will divide. From eight to ninety-six buds, and every bud will grow into a perfectly formed embryo, and every embryo into a full-sized adult. Making ninety-six human beings grow where only one grew before. Progress ...

Identical twins – but not in the piddling twos and threes as in the old viviparous days, when an egg would sometimes accidentally divide; actually by dozens, by scores at a time.

'Scores', the Director repeated and flung out his arms, as though he were distributing largesse. 'Scores.'

But one of the students was fool enough to ask where the advantage lay.

'My good boy!' The Director wheeled sharply round on him. 'Can't you see? Can't you *see*?' He raised a hand; his expression was solemn. 'Bokanovsky's Process is one of the major instruments of social stability!'

Major instruments of social stability.

Standard men and women; in uniform batches. The whole of a small factory staffed with the products of a single bokanovskified egg.

'Ninety-six identical twins working ninety-six identical machines!' The voice was almost tremulous with enthusiasm. 'You really know where you are. For the first time in history.' He quoted the planetary motto. 'Community, Identity, Stability.' Grand words. 'If we could bokanovskify indefinitely the whole problem would be solved.'

Solved by standard Gammas, unvarying Deltas, uniform Epsilons. Millions of identical twins. The principle of mass production at last applied to biology.

Aldous Huxley (1932) Brave New World

CASE STUDY 10.3

2374 Couples who discover that they are sterile suffer greatly. 'What will you give me', asks Abraham of God, 'for I continue childless?' And Rachel cries to her husband Jacob, 'Give me children, or I shall die!'

2375 Research aimed at reducing human sterility is to be encouraged, on condition that it is placed 'at the service of the human person, of his inalienable rights, and his true and integral good according to the design and will of God.'

2376 Techniques that entail the dissociation of husband and wife, by the intrusion of a person other than the couple (donation of sperm or ovum, surrogate uterus), are gravely immoral. These techniques (heterologous artificial insemination and fertilization) infringe the child's right to be born of a father and mother known to him and bound to each other by marriage. They betray the spouses' 'right to become a father and a mother only through each other.'

2377 Techniques involving only the married couple (homologous artificial insemination and fertilization) are perhaps less reprehensible, yet remain morally unacceptable. They dissociate the sexual act from the procreative act. The act which brings the child into existence is no longer an act by which two persons give themselves to one another, but one that 'entrusts the life and identity of the embryo into the power of doctors and biologists and establishes the domination of technology over the origin and destiny of the human person. Such a relationship of domination is in itself contrary to the dignity and equality that must be common to parents and children.' 'Under the moral aspect procreation is deprived of its proper perfection when it is not willed as the fruit of the conjugal act, that is to say, of the specific act of the spouses' union … Only respect for the link between the meanings of the conjugal act and respect for the unity of the human being make possible procreation in conformity with the dignity of the person.'

2378 A child is not something owed to one, but is a gift. The 'supreme gift of marriage' is a human person. A child may not be considered a piece of property, an idea to which an alleged 'right to a child' would lead. In this area, only the child possesses genuine rights: the right 'to be the fruit of the specific act of the conjugal love of his parents', and 'the right to be respected as a person from the moment of his conception.'

'Catechism of the Catholic Church', Pt III 'Life in Christ'

Ian Wilmut, the scientist who led the team behind Dolly the sheep, launched a passionate attack yesterday on plans to clone humans, saying it would be 'extremely cruel' for the mothers and resultant children.

In an article in the US journal *Science*, Dr Wilmut denounced the declared aim of the Italian and US fertility specialists Severino Antinori and Panos Zavos to clone humans and enable infertile men to pass on their genes.

In language a world away from the optimism in 1997 at the birth of Dolly, Dr Wilmut warned that four years of experiments on animals had shown the cloning technique to be deeply flawed, exacting a huge toll of miscarriages and deformities.

'There is no reason to believe that the outcomes of attempted human cloning will be any different', he wrote.

Since Dolly, scientists have cloned mice, cattle, goats and pigs. Dr Wilmut and Dr Jaenisch point out that very few cloned embryos survive to birth and many of these die shortly after. Survivors are often grotesquely large or have defects ...

Dr Wilmut ... said he thought that another quantum leap, as great as that to create Dolly, was needed to make cloning reliable. That might take 50 years. Even then he would oppose human cloning, on social and ethical grounds.

'A parent of a cloned child would be much more likely than usual to impose their expectations and limitations on the child, because they'll think: "This child is like me, therefore I know how it's going to behave." David Beckham's son, Brooklyn, may be under a lot of pressure to become a footballer. But if he was genetically identical to his father, that pressure would be even greater.'

James Meek (2001) 'Dolly's creator says no to human cloning', *Guardian Unlimited*, 29 March

CASE STUDY 10.5

Pre-implantation genetic diagnosis (PGD) is a technique that involves the use of assisted reproduction technology. A woman's ovaries are stimulated through hormones to enable the collection of a number of eggs, which are then fertilised in the laboratory with sperm. Fertilised eggs are allowed to divide and multiply for 3–5 days, by which stage they contain about eight cells or a blastocyst.

At this stage one or two cells are removed for testing. A large number of undesirable genetic conditions (such as muscular dystrophy) can be identified through this testing – as can the gender of the embryo. On the basis of these tests a decision is made as to which, if any, of the embryos will be transplanted into the mother's uterus.

Provided by the authors

CASE STUDY 10.6

Stephen is the child I have been attempting to conceive for the past seventeen years. Stephen is why Toby and I are involved in the IVF programme. Stephen is waiting inside my mind. His spirit lives inside me and waits for nature or my doctors to form his body – the body that will set him free to live. Only once in all my years as a midwife, I held a baby girl in my arms; she was the exact image of Stephen. So in real life I have held my dreamtime child in my arms, touched him, fed him, and looked after him. I know him. He began in me …

When I was twenty-one I started my attempt at pregnancy and began to realize that things were not going to be easy. Eventually, I had five years of very painful investigations and tubal treatments. The two major operations to repair my damaged Fallopian tubes only resulted in two ectopic pregnancies. Further repair work on what was left of my remaining tube was a waste of time. All my treatments were at considerable cost to myself and the community …

Toby and I have been on the IVF programme in Melbourne since 1978 … Is it right for us to want a child when my body would no longer be able to conceive children naturally? Since we have always felt particularly fertile and have always wanted our child, we have always considered that we had as much right to choose children as any of our more fertile friends. In some respects our child has already chosen us. You don't suddenly stop wanting a child because of some physical problem. If you suddenly became blind in an accident, would you turn to your children and say, 'We don't want you now because we cannot see you'? It's the same for couples with an infertility problem because we can't see our children it doesn't stop them from being there. Like blind parents we can still feel our children's presence.

William AW Walters and Peter Singer (eds) (1982) *Test-Tube Babies*

A woman of 58 is to become one of Britain's oldest mothers after having fertility treatment at a controversial private clinic, it emerged yesterday.

Ian Craft, director of the London Fertility Centre, said he was 'delighted' that his patient, known as Sandra, was to give birth shortly. Her age indicates that she became pregnant via egg donation. Her case satisfied the criteria laid down by the human fertilisation and embryology authority.

Sandra is the third woman over 55 to hit the headlines following treatment at the clinic, thought to be the only unit in the UK helping women of that age.

In 1997, a Welsh hill farmer Liz Buttle, 60, became the oldest mother in Britain after lying about her age to receive treatment. Two years ago Lynne Bezant, 56, and her husband Derek, 55, had twins following treatment at the clinic. Other units have lower age limits, usually about 50, and most health authorities do not fund treatment for women over 36.

'I think we should be encouraging responsible practice in the UK, which would be to confine treatment to women below the age of menopause', said Richard Kennedy, secretary of the British Fertility Society ...

The HFEA [Human Fertilisation and Embryology Authority], which regulates fertility treatment, does not specify an upper age limit for assisted conception. But it states that a couple's health, ages and 'likely future ability to look after or provide for a child's needs' should be considered by the ethics committees which decide whether clinics can treat patients.

The world's oldest mother is thought to be Rosanna Dalla Corta, from Italy, who gave birth in 1994 at the age of 63.

Tania Branigan (2003) 'Woman, 58, set to give birth',
The Guardian, 29 January

ETHICS IN PRACTICE

Michelle and Jayson Whitaker, from Bicester, near Oxford, had asked the Human Fertilisation and Embryology Authority (HFEA) to approve a licence allowing doctors to use a 'tissue-typing' IVF technique, which would have provided a perfect tissue match for their three-year-old son Charlie.

Charlie suffers from a rare blood disorder, Diamond Blackfan anaemia (DBA), and must undergo painful daylong blood transfusion and daily injections of life-saving drugs. The licence would have enabled the child, who is critically ill, to have a potentially life-saving bone marrow transplant.

But the HFEA ruled it could not approve the procedure as it would be unethical and would break the law on human fertilisation and embryology.

'Every member of the authority on the committee had enormous sympathy for Charlie Whitaker and his parents, but they were unable to approve the licence', an HFEA spokeswoman said.

The Whitakers wanted their doctor, Dr Mohammed Tarranissi, to be allowed to test embryos taken from Mrs Whitaker using a procedure called pre-implantation genetic diagnosis, PGD. This is normally done for couples, one or both of whom carry a genetic disorder.

Through PGD the doctors can examine the embryos to make sure the one selected for implantation in the mother does not carry the inherited genetic disorder. But in the Whitakers' case, Charlie's disorder is 'sporadic', meaning the chances of his parents having another baby with the disease is no greater than with the general public – between five and seven per million live births.

So there is no reason to believe Mrs Whitaker's embryos would again hold the genetic disorder affecting Charlie.

The Whitakers wanted the doctors to be allowed, or licensed, to check the embryos so they could choose one that would provide a perfect tissue match for Charlie. Charlie's little brother or sister would then be able to donate bone-marrow, potentially saving the youngster's life.

The special cells would help Charlie's body create red blood cells and give him a 90% chance of recovery. But a transplant must be carried out within 18 months to have a good chance of success.

However, the HFEA said that under the 1990 Human Fertilisation and Embryology Act, it is unable to licence the 'tissue typing' procedure. It is the first time such an application has been made.

It said the procedure the Whitakers want to carry out would not be to check whether the embryos carried a genetic disorder, but to see whether the embryo was a match for Charlie.

The couple have denied they are creating a 'designer' baby, as they are not choosing the baby's sex, intelligence or skin colour. But the HFEA has argued that the procedure would mean selecting one life, or embryo, which matches Charlie's tissue type, over another life, another embryo, which does not.

The organisation claims that the public is happy with the procedure of checking embryos to ensure they are free of genetic disorders, but does not support using the procedure to check embryos for other reasons, including tissue typing.

Rebecca Allison (2002) 'New designer baby row as watchdog rejects family's plea for treatment', The Guardian, 2 August

ETHICAL ANALYSIS

Human reproduction is simultaneously a natural process and deeply culturally influenced. Every society that we know of has highly developed norms regulating the relations between the sexes, and the rearing of children. Western societies have seen a good deal of liberalisation in these matters, as in many others, over the past few decades. Until quite recently, for example, the stigma associated with children born out of wedlock – bastards – forced many unmarried mothers to give their children up for adoption. Only in the past few decades have we seen the abolition of the legal discrimination against such children, which meant they did not have the same claims on their parents' estate as children born in wedlock.

Strong legal and moral prohibitions remain, of course, in relation to sexual relations with children, and between family members. Many people also disapprove of sexual relations between people of very different ages and, in some cases, even of relations between members of different religious, racial or ethnic groups. However, there is broad acceptance of the existence of procreative rights. While there is now general agreement that everyone has a right not to be forced to become parents against their will, nor to have their reproductive capacity destroyed against their will (see case study 10.1) there is little agreement about what else such rights imply. There is, for example, dispute as to who is morally entitled to reproduce. Some argue that all competent adults have such a right; others that it belongs only to (heterosexual) married couples. There are also fundamental disagreements about what people may do to control their fertility (as demonstrated in the on-going debates about contraception and, especially, abortion), as well as disagreements about what they may do to enhance it. Issues around the enhancement of fertility have arisen as a consequence of the development of Assisted Reproductive Technology (ART). We will turn our attention to some of the controversies that ART has generated below. To inform our discussion, however, we first focus more closely on the nature of procreative rights.

Procreative rights

Discussions of procreative rights – rights to bear and raise children – are always going to be complicated, because they involve the interests of three different groups:

- (potential) parents;
- (potential) offspring;
- society.

Each group's interests may be different from the other. It is (potential) parents, who have (or lack) procreative rights. To understand the nature of these rights we need to notice a distinction between two kinds of rights: 'liberty' rights, and 'claim' rights. Let us look first at liberty rights. Often to say that we have a right to something, or to act in a certain way, is simply to say that we do no wrong in so acting, and so others should not prevent us doing so. You have a right, for example, to walk down the street on your hands. If you feel like doing this, and you are able to do so, others ought not prevent you from indulging your whim. You have a right – a liberty right – to do it. On other occasions to say that we have a right does not simply imply that others should not interfere with us if we try to gain the object of the right, but rather that they should actively assist us in gaining it; we can 'claim' the object of the right from them. Think for example of the right to primary education. To say that children have such a right is not simply to say that they (or their parents) do no wrong if they try to obtain a primary school education. Rather, it implies that others (the state, say, or the community) should provide such an education through, for example, the funding of accessible primary schools. In societies such as Australia, then, the right to primary education is clearly understood as a claim right. Generally, of course, it will be easier to support assertions of liberty rights than those of claim rights, since liberty rights only require that others do not interfere with the activities of the right holder, while claim rights impose active duties to assist on others.

Procreative rights seem in the first place to be, or to follow from, liberty rights. In liberal societies such as Australia, it is generally accepted that, provided we are not interfering with others against their wishes, or behaving in ways which will have seriously bad consequences, we have a right to be left alone and to do as we wish with our bodies, including engaging in consensual sexual activity. Since we have a (liberty) right to such activity, and reproduction is a predictable outcome of it, it would seem to follow that we also have a right to procreate. Furthermore, limiting procreative rights – at least over unassisted reproduction – could only be enforced through particularly gross intrusions into an important part of people's private lives.

These are negative reasons why we should accept the existence of a liberty right to procreate. But there are also powerful positive reasons why we should grant people such a right. Most people grow up in a family setting and many have strong desires to create a family of their own, and to have genetic offspring (for an expression of the strength of such a desire see case study 10.6). It is unsurprising that an urge to parent should be felt by many, since the urge to procreate and special concern for one's offspring seem to be based in our animal nature. Furthermore, we are usually on the end, as it were, of a chain of family relations, and it seems reasonable to want – and perhaps even to feel obliged – to continue that. Many people, then, see reproduction as a great good, something they aim to achieve. That people have an interest in being able to procreate is a reason to grant them the right to do so.

If our reproductive choices had no impact on others, then, it would seem that people should be allowed to procreate as, and when, they pleased. But of course those choices do affect others, in the first place the children who are brought into existence as a result of that choice. What considerations relevant to the interests of their (potential) children should weigh with (potential) parents in deciding whether they should or should not procreate? One principle that plausibly can be appealed to here is what we'll call the 'worthwhile life principle', viz: 'Don't create people who will (or are likely to) have lives that are not worth living.'

Few would disagree with this, though of course what makes a life worth living is far from straightforward. Some people who labour under great physical or social handicaps clearly obtain much joy from their life. Others who appear blessed by good fortune feel their existence is a burden. Nevertheless, being born into an environment of severe material deprivation or emotional turmoil, or with a painful degenerative condition, are clearly factors which are likely to make it difficult to have a life that is worth living. For just such reasons, people often try to avoid having children who will be so affected. On the other hand, if the children who are brought into being will (probably) have lives that are worth living, then it appears that their parents have done no wrong to them in procreating; indeed, they should be grateful to their parents for giving them life. In any case, provided the worthwhile life principle is satisfied, then considerations of the welfare of children to be brought into being seem compatible with the existence of a broad procreative right.

The decision to have (or not have) children also affects the community at large, which will bear many of the costs associated with educating and caring for them, and which will benefit from their work and contributions later in life. Indeed, many countries have population policies, aiming to restrict the number of children born (as in China and India), or to increase it (as in Australia). In non-authoritarian countries, at least, such policies work through the provision of incentives rather than legal requirements. They are, then, compatible with the recognition of procreative rights.

Assisted Reproductive Technology (ART)

In recent years huge advances in scientific knowledge of, and technological control over, human reproduction have occurred. Much of this has been driven by progress in plant and animal husbandry, via selective breeding and, for just over a hundred years, scientific breeding based on an understanding of genetics. The development of Assisted Reproductive Technology (ART) for humans has opened up two broad fields of possibilities, both of which are fraught with moral difficulties.

Firstly, ART allows many people who could not previously procreate for either physical reasons (because they are infertile, or past menopause, for example) or for social reasons (because they are in an exclusive lesbian relationship, say) to be able to do so. The original 'test tube baby' (Louise Brown), born in 1978, was the first child conceived outside a human body; now thousands of women a year have babies conceived through in-vitro fertilisation (IVF). ('*In Vitro*' is a Latin term that literally means 'in glass': IVF fertilisation involves removing a woman's eggs and fertilising them in a laboratory, then reimplanting the fertilised eggs in the womb.) The cloning of Dolly the sheep in 1997 demonstrated that we now have the means to reproduce animals asexually. The unreliability of the technique of reproductive cloning at this point in time makes it unthinkable for human use (see case study 10.4).

Secondly, ART is giving us much greater control over the kinds of children we have. Our increased knowledge of genetics, especially the discovery of DNA and the mapping of the human genome, mean that decisions as to which of the fertilised IVF embryos should be implanted in a woman's womb can be based on information about their genetic make-up gained through techniques such as pre-implantation genetic diagnosis (PGD). And as our knowledge of genetics improves, it seems likely that rather than simply having to accept the genetic make-up of such embryos, we will be able to 'genetically engineer' them to cause them to have desired properties.

These developments have generated much ethical controversy. At one extreme are those who are absolutely opposed to any use of ART. The official Catholic position (see case study 10.3) is that the only morally legitimate means to reproduction is sexual intercourse between a husband and wife, and that we must not prevent a pregnancy proceeding naturally: it follows that all ART is morally unacceptable (Finnis (1980) contains a sophisticated explication and defence of the Catholic view on sexual morality.) At the other extreme are those who see ART as either, in itself, morally unproblematic, simply another medical technology that should be made available to any competent adult who wishes to make use of it, or even as generally morally good, allowing us for the first time to start to take control of human reproduction, rather than being at the mercy of unpredictable natural processes. Others have a more nuanced view, seeing certain forms of ART (such as IVF) as acceptable, at least in certain circumstances, and others (especially reproductive cloning) as always bad. This view probably has most popular support, and is reflected in legislation in most jurisdictions. The state either heavily regulates such technologies as IVF, laying down strict rules about who may gain access to them and in what circumstances (see case studies 10.7 and 10.8), or totally outlaws them (as is the case with reproductive cloning).

Some of the opposition to ART appears to be based more on a mistrust of new developments than reasoned argument (Bostrom and Ord 2006). If this is true, as people become more accustomed to the different kinds of ART, they will (most likely) find them less morally objectionable. This is in fact what has happened with IVF, which attracted widespread opposition when first used, but now, according to surveys, is widely approved of as a treatment for infertility. Other opposition is based on certain religious commitments. Whatever the ultimate status of such commitments, they obviously cannot be used as the basis for public policy or moral consensus in a religiously pluralist society. That said, there are well articulated arguments both against and for ART, either in general, or in particular cases. We now turn to a consideration of these arguments.

ART and reproduction

First, we consider the issues around the use of ART to allow those who have been unable to procreate to do so. As we indicated above, there is general acceptance that people have a liberty right to procreate naturally. However, there is obviously much less agreement about whether, and under what circumstances, people have a right to use artificial means to procreate. Here we can distinguish between assertions that there are liberty rights to use the various forms of ART, and assertions that there are claim rights to them. As we said above, it is generally easier to justify assertions of liberty rights than assertions of claim rights. We also saw that there are two kinds of reasons in favour of accepting a liberty right to natural procreation: we are entitled to do what we want with our bodies; and people place great value on being able to have genetic offspring. Both these reasons obviously also apply to those who seek to use ART. So, on the face of it, if there is a general liberty right to procreate, there is a liberty right to procreate using ART. That is, if people wish to use ART and can find medical practitioners who will help them do so, they should not be prevented from doing so.

However, there are arguably important differences between natural reproduction and assisted reproduction that make the supposed liberty right to use ART less secure than the general right to procreate. Natural reproduction involves sexual activity, so any attempt to constrain it necessarily involves interference in a deeply personal activity. There is good reason to be wary of the state surveillance and invasion of private life that would be necessary to enforce such constraint. Restrictions on ART, on the other hand, simply deny access to a technology, so do not involve any such interference in personal activities or invasion of private space.

Still, even if we accept that these important differences between natural and assisted reproduction exist, they do not themselves show that there is not a liberty right to ART for reproductive purposes. At most, they may become relevant to that claim if there are other reasons to hold that assisted reproduction is undesirable in ways that natural reproduction is not. As we will see below, this is exactly what opponents of ART do claim.

Before turning to those issues, however, we should consider the proposition that people (sometimes) have a claim right to ART. The research that leads to progress in ART is expensive (consider the obstacles that stand in the way of bringing the techniques of reproductive cloning to the point where they are safe to be used by humans, for example). Furthermore, access to ART for prospective parents is also costly. Does society have a duty to invest in ART research? Does it have a duty to subsidise those who would otherwise be denied access to it through lack of financial means?

These questions are open even for those who accept that there is a liberty right to ART. The answer that is given to them will depend at least in part on how conditions such as infertility are characterised. Some think that infertility should be seen as a serious medical condition, like being a paraplegic, which restricts one's chances to live a normal life. In our society, those who suffer from disabling medical conditions are usually provided with help to enable them to live in a more normal way. So if infertility is a disabling medical condition, it seems only fair that those who suffer from it should also be assisted to overcome it.

Others think that infertility should be seen as falling within the normal range of human variation. No doubt some infertile people will prefer not to be infertile, just as some redheads would prefer to have a complexion that was better suited to Australian conditions, and some unattractive people wish they were better looking. That is, infertility is at most a misfortune, but not a disease or disability. We don't generally think we have to provide assistance to people who suffer from such misfortunes. So we are not being unfair in not providing assistance to the infertile to overcome their misfortune.

There are clearly reasons to allow people to use ART for reproduction, since it enables them to have the offspring they wish for, but could not otherwise have. On the other hand, it has been claimed that considerations of the welfare of the children who would be born as the result of the use of ART weigh against allowing it, in some or even all cases. Such arguments have been very influential in the widespread opposition to reproductive cloning (see case study 10.4), as well as in support of restricting access to less controversial methods of reproductive ART, such as IVF.

We cannot go into the whole range of arguments that support ART's restriction or even total prohibition. However, some of these arguments have a shared defect. Let us consider the case in Victoria. Until a few years ago, this state legally prohibited single women from access to IVF. Supporters of the legislation claimed that children of single women tend to be disadvantaged relative to children of couples. Therefore they felt that legislation preventing single women gaining access to IVF was justified, on the grounds of the relative welfare of children. Similarly, opponents of legalising reproductive cloning, even if it becomes safe, claim that the presumed genetic identity of the cloned child with their parent will lead to greater expectations that they will live up to the achievements of their parent. This will be much more burdensome than is the case with naturally conceived children. (See case study 10.4.) So reproductive cloning should be legally prohibited, again on grounds of relative welfare.

Such arguments have a common form. Firstly, they point to the (supposed) difference in welfare between members of two groups of children. Then, on the basis of this, they conclude that due to concern for the welfare of children, potential parents of children who would belong to the less well-off group should be denied access to the ART which would enable them to bring such children into being. Even if we accept the claims about the relative welfare of the different groups of children, the conclusion does not follow. To see why, we need to look more closely at the appeal to the welfare of the (potential) children on which the conclusion is supposedly grounded.

We have discussed one principle relevant to the welfare of potential children in our consideration of procreative rights above, what we called the 'worthwhile life principle', viz: 'Don't create people who will (or are likely to) have lives that are not worth living.' Deciding whether the use of ART satisfies this principle does not involve any comparative judgments. Provided that a child is likely to have a life that is worth living, then the principle is satisfied. Since it is not suggested that, for example, children of single mothers do not usually have lives worth living (at least not in virtue of being children of single mothers) then it would seem that allowing access to ART cannot be ruled out by appeal to this principle. The fact (if it is a fact) that such children will have a lower level of welfare than that of children in other groups, does not show that they are harmed by being brought into existence. Much less does it show that children have a right to two parents (a claim made by the former Australian Prime Minister John Howard). Indeed, if we accepted that whether or not potential parents have a right to procreate should be determined according to the relative welfare of the children they might bear, many people who currently uncontroversially possess such a right would have it stripped from them, for example, economically disadvantaged people. (This is just what the eugenics movement, discussed in case study 10.1, proposed, of course, and at least in part it did so for these types of reasons.)

The reason why appeals to the welfare of children who would be born if ART were generally accessible have been so influential as grounds for restricting such access is, of course, a matter of speculation. But at least in part, it may reflect a certain common confusion about the nature of potential children. A principle which is relevant in making decisions about how to treat *children* is what we will call the 'greater welfare' principle, viz 'When a decision has to be made between a number of options available for a child, choose the one which will (probably) produce the greatest increase in welfare for the child.'

Say, for example, we are deciding whether to send a child to a single-sex or coeducational school. We look at evidence that suggests that one of these settings correlates with greater on-going subjective well-being, as well as academic and financial success, and so on. Then we decide that this is obviously a very good reason to prefer that setting. It might be tempting to think along the following lines.

If a potential child is born into a two-parent family their welfare is likely to be greater than if they are born into a single-parent family. Therefore, in accordance with the greater welfare principle, we should ensure that they are born into the two-parent family.

So the greater welfare principle might seem to tell us that potential children should be born to parents who are likely to provide the conditions in which they will live a life of greater welfare. Such reasoning rests on mistakenly applying the greater welfare principle to potential children. From the fact that this principle can reasonably be applied to actual children in certain contexts, it does not follow that it ought to be applied to potential children, or indeed can be applied to them. We suggest that it cannot. To see this let us first get it clear what we mean when we speak of potential children. Generally, when we add some descriptor (such as 'unpleasant' or 'tall') to the word 'children', it picks out actual children (all those who are tall, for example). 'Potential', however, does not work like this. Potential children are no more children than wooden horses are horses. We should not think of potential children as existing entities inhabiting some ghostly region waiting to be assigned to the people who will become their parents. When we speak of potential children we are talking of what might come to pass, not what is. At one time each of us was, so to speak, a potential child. But we were only the potential child of the people who are actually our parents.

As we have seen, the welfare principle applies to actual children, at least in certain contexts. That is, sometimes we should seek to remove comparative disadvantages between actual children. However, the welfare principle does not apply to potential children, since the issue of whether or not to make a potential child actual is not a comparative issue to be resolved by determining and redressing inequalities between two or more sets of potential children, or between sets of potential children and sets of actual children. Rather, to reiterate, the issue is whether or not one or more potential children ought to be made actual. No doubt some potential children, for example, children without brains, should not be allowed to be made actual. However, the threshold set of properties that ought to determine the eligibility of a potential child to be an actual child ought not to be confused with the possible need to redress comparative disadvantage among actual children; these are simply different issues. Specifically, potential children can meet a reasonable eligibility test for being made actual even though, once actual, they are significantly disadvantaged relative to other actual children. Here again, consider the potential children of economically disadvantaged parents. Hence, we cannot appeal to the 'greater welfare' principle to justify restricting access to ART.

ART and choosing children

As ART is giving us new ways of conceiving children, it is also giving us greater control over the kind of children we have. Pre-implantation genetic diagnosis (PGD) allows us to decide which of the fertilised embryos available for implantation in IVF is to be used on the basis of their genetic make-up. And our growing knowledge of 'genetic engineering' will increasingly allow us to change the genetic make-up of embryos, either before they are implanted in IVF, or even in utero. These developments open up radically new possibilities. Previously we only possessed the capacity to decide whether or not we had children; these new techniques are increasingly giving us the power to determine the nature of the children we will have. We now can reach, as it were, into the first nine months of life to shape our children in a way which has never been possible before.

Some of the applications of this power seem relatively uncontroversial. As indicated in case studies 10.5 and 10.8 it is broadly accepted that we are morally permitted to use techniques such as PGD to 'screen out' IVF embryos that carry debilitating genetic conditions such as muscular dystrophy. This is, in fact, an application of the 'worthwhile life' principle discussed above.

Other applications, however, are much more controversial. Should we be allowed, for instance, to use such techniques not simply to prevent the birth of children who will probably not have lives worth living, but also to select – or create – children who are desirable for other reasons? (See the discussions in Savulescu and Bostrom (2008).) The *Brave New World* scenario described in case study 10.2, where a race of identical willing drones can be created, illustrates the potential for abuse that this exercise could open up.

The *Brave New World* scenario, however, pictures a world in which the desired qualities to implant in a child are those which benefit *other* people. Would it not be acceptable – even good – to provide children with qualities which will make life better for *them*? Imagine a parent selecting one embryo over another because the first will grow up to be a calmer, or smarter, person than the second (assuming there is sufficient scientific basis for such a choice). Having a calm rather than anxious temperament seems to be good both for the person who possesses it and for those around them.

Attractive as this idea might be, it is also not without problems. Consider that in many parts of the world being born female is a serious disadvantage relative to being born male. (And in fact prenatal testing for gender is relatively widespread, and abortion on basis of sex relatively common, in such places.) The parent who aims to choose the qualities which are likely to make the life of their future child better should, then, select for a male rather than female child. In so doing, however, they become at least complicit with morally iniquitous sexist attitudes and practices. Indeed, such a person may be more than simply complicit, they may actually be perpetuating and reinforcing those attitudes and practices. In choosing to implant an embryo on the grounds that it is a boy rather than a girl, they are in effect sending a message that being female is a bad thing, to be avoided if possible.

Moreover, the attempt to select for qualities which give our child a relative advantage may, in some cases, be both self-defeating, and socially undesirable (Schelling 1978). In a sexist society, it is currently an advantage to be male. But consider the likely consequences if many parents choose to have boy children rather than girls, producing a large preponderance of males. Firstly, given the scarcity of women, it might actually be advantageous to be female, with each woman having her choice among a number of possible marriage partners. Secondly, many of the males will find themselves without a marriage partner of any kind. Surely, such a society is not to be desired. (Evidence suggests that China is heading in this direction as a result of its 'single child' policy.)

The difficult ethical issues raised by our new power to shape the kind of children we give birth to may become more tractable if we notice that that power is actually an extension of the ability we already have to shape and influence children once born. Though the particular problems raised are novel, many of them, at least, are of a kind with which we are already familiar. Consider the case we just looked at of the parent faced with making a choice that appears to be to the advantage of their child, but which will reinforce a morally bad state of affairs. This is analogous to the situation of a well-to-do parent who believes in equality of opportunity for children and has to choose between sending their child to an overcrowded and under-resourced government school, or paying for a place in a well equipped exclusive private school. In both cases, the difficulties arise because a choice has to be made in a situation that is already morally imperfect, generating a conflict between the action that is most beneficial for a loved one, and the action that will be most in keeping with our broader moral values. Even the *Brave New World* scenario is not unfamiliar. In a society organised along class lines, the reality is that many people will be shaped in ways that fit them to accept their positions as relatively menial workers. Indeed, Aldous Huxley, the author of *Brave New World*, clearly intended that book not simply as a description of a possible world, but as an allegory illuminating the dangerous tendencies that he believed already existed in the society of his time.

Seeing how the problems created by ART can be understood as instances of common moral difficulties does not necessarily make them any easier to deal with. It may, however, lead us to think that though ART produces new instances of such difficulties, in itself it is not a morally problematic matter. Some believe, on the other hand, that ART *is* morally problematic in itself (Kass 2002). Until now, human reproduction has involved *begetting* children, where we cause a pregnancy, but have no control over the nature of the child that issues from that pregnancy. Begetting, then, has forced us to confront and accommodate risk, diversity and difference in the process which is at the heart of the continuation of the human species. When we use ART, by contrast, we *make* children: not only do we cause a pregnancy, but we control the outcome of that pregnancy. Increasingly, the process of reproduction is tending to a form of manufacturing, in which we can minimise risk and remove unwanted difference and diversity in the children we produce. Those who express these concerns worry that ART is bringing about fundamental changes in our attitude to the reproductive process; changes that will in turn impact on what it is to be human and our understanding thereof.

Readings

Allison, Rebecca (2002) 'New designer baby row as watchdog rejects family's plea for treatment', *The Guardian*, 2 August, available at <http://www.guardian.co.uk> (accessed 23/1/09).

Black, Edwin (2003) 'The horrifying American roots of Nazi eugenics', *History News Network*, 24 November, available at <http://hnn.us/articles/1796.html> (accessed 23/1/09).

Bostrom, Nick and Ord, Toby (2006) 'The reversal test: Eliminating status quo bias in applied ethics', *Ethics*, vol 116, no 4, July, pp 656–79.

Branigan, Tania (2003) 'Woman, 58, set to give birth', *The Guardian*, 29 January, available at <http://www.guardian.co.uk> (accessed 23/1/09).

Burley, Justine and Harris, John (eds) (2002) *Blackwell Companion to Genetics*, Blackwell, Oxford.

'Catechism of the Catholic Church', Pt III 'Life in Christ, The gift of a child', available at <http://www.vatican.va/archive/catechism/p3s2c2a6.htm I> (accessed 23/1/09).

Finnis, John (1980) *Natural Law and Natural Rights*, Oxford University Press, Oxford.

Huxley, Aldous (1932) *Brave New World*, Chatto & Windus, London, pp 10–11.

Kass, Leon R (2002) *Life, Liberty, and the Defense of Dignity*, Encounter Books, New York.

Meek, James (2001) 'Dolly's creator says no to human cloning', *Guardian Unlimited*,

29 March, available at <http://www.guardian.co.uk> (accessed 23/1/09).

Oderberg, David (2000) *Applied Ethics: A Non-consequentialist Approach*, Blackwell, Oxford.

Savulescu, Julian and Bostrom, Nick (eds) (2008) *Enhancement of Human Beings*, Oxford University Press, Oxford.

Schelling, Thomas (1978) 'Choosing our children's genes' in Schelling, Thomas (1978) *Micromotives and Macrobehaviour*, Norton, New York.

Singer, Peter and Kuhse, Helga (eds) (2000) *Blackwell Companion to Bioethics*, Blackwell, Oxford.

Walters, William and Singer, Peter (eds) (1982) *Test-Tube Babies*, Oxford University Press, Melbourne, pp 120–21.

11: The institution of the family

Olive is an elderly woman who lives with her adult son Robert who has an intellectual disability. Part of this disability involves epilepsy, which is controlled by medication twice per day. Olive has developed cancer and has been given months to live. She relies on her son to look after at home, carry the shopping etc. Staff at the local day care centre where Robert attends notice that his appearance is deteriorating. He is losing weight, his personal hygiene has declined and his clothes are dirty. Robert has also had some fits while at day care. Previously they have been well controlled.

The staff contact the social worker Janet, asking her to find permanent accommodation for Robert where he will be well looked after. Janet knows that there is no accommodation close by and that Robert would have to leave the area if he is to be placed somewhere. Olive has no transport and perhaps Olive and Robert would not be able to see each other if he was moved.

When she visits Olive to discuss Robert's situation, Janet finds that Olive is adamant that she and Robert are managing well. Olive is teary and loud in her condemnation of 'interfering busybodies at day care'. She says that she has a good mind to keep Robert at home away from their influence altogether, but she does need the break and he enjoys his days there. As to leaving home, Olive points out that Robert is all she has and she is all he has and that they should be left in peace to see out her last few months. They have the right to continue in their own home as long as possible, she says. It is not clear what Robert wants.

Provided by Wendy Bowles

CASE STUDY 11.2

Bridgette rings Douglas, a family therapist, to make an appointment for some counselling for her whole family. She says the appointment has been made to discuss the children's poor behaviour. They have no respect for their parents, particularly her, and she feels she can no longer go on without some help. The appointment is attended by Tony, the husband, Bridgette, Bill the 18-year-old son, Sally the 16-year-old daughter and Scott the 13-year-old son.

During the interview it becomes apparent that Tony and the children believe that they are there to discuss the mother's depression and headaches. No mention is made of the young peoples' behaviour nor their so-called lack of respect by Bridgette. When Douglas asks if there is anything else that the family would like to discuss apart from Bridgette's headaches and depression there is silence. Bridgette looks down and twists her handkerchief.

Provided by Wendy Bowles

CASE STUDY 11.3

She was little short of beautiful; without make-up, thick, heavy dark hair in a bob, pale delicate skin, dark tear-wet lashes, sporting the beginnings of a shiner. Slight, small and heavily pregnant, she held herself with poise and there wasn't a man in the 2 am Sunday quiet of the charge room at North Sydney police station whose sympathies were not instantly engaged as, in faltering English, she stumbled through her story. Recently arrived German immigrants, things hadn't gone well for her and Manny. This, their first child, was arriving to familial stress and economic uncertainty; an enterprise begun in hope was foundering and Manny, her husband, the only person she knew in Australia, in frustration and despair, turned on her and physically abused her. They had a little flat in Mount Street at the rear of the police station and she had run from it, seeking help.

This was a matter in which the police could positively take action, they would arrest the abuser; there was an immediate gathering up of torches and batons, caps and truck keys. From her look of dawning horror, this wasn't at all what the young wife wanted. She didn't want Manny charged; after tears and explanations it came out that what she wanted was the young man she married back. That being beyond the ability of police, the best they could offer was safety; they would instantly remove him from the family home. She wavered, then gathering resolve, shook her head and left the station, determined to preserve her marriage. No, she didn't want the police to speak to Manny, not now; that threat to her marriage had to be kept away.

She was back in a half-hour, stumbling awkwardly in through the charge room door, blubbering wordlessly like a child. Blood streamed down her shins, where Manny had been kicking her. They took her to the muster room where she laid her head on her crossed arms on the table and sobbed as if her heart would break. The truck crew left to arrest her husband.

Manny was a surprise; instead of a Teutonic brute with a blonde crew-cut and no back to his head, he was small and slight, dark haired, pale and quite good looking; his wife and he might easily pass for brother and sister. Standing in the dock in the charge room, positively rigid with rage, he declined to answer questions or supply information. The wife was brought through to sign the charge book, then to be taken to the casualty ward. She wilted at the sight of Manny in the dock. When the charge book was proffered for her signature, she asked Manny what should she do? He refused to answer, would not even look at her. She walked over to the dock and spoke again and in a graceful and infinitely appealing gesture, she reached out and touched his chin, to draw his face towards her; Manny's response was a vicious punch, aimed at her face.

Intercepted by a beefy shoulder, a sergeant quickly moved in; a backhander drove Manny to the far end of the dock, face livid with fingermarks as his wife was bustled out. Legs bandaged, she was back before breakfast-time, with toothbrush and toiletries for Manny, which he hurled away, across his cell. He remained there, determined and furious, bail-refused, until Monday morning.

In its crudity and narrow focus, civil libertarian law reform provides means-tested legal representation for defendants, but ignores their unrepresented victims. The public solicitor told Manny what to do and Manny gave directions to his wife at five minutes to ten, in a few, savagely barked commands; when called, she informed the Magistrate she did not now want to proceed with the prosecution and Manny was discharged. Last seen, she was running behind Manny on the Pacific Highway, trying to speak to him as he strode manfully from the court. One of the arresting police said, 'At least we kept her safe for one night' which described the police task accurately. It wasn't to secure a conviction, they understood that she would withdraw proceedings against her husband. It wasn't to resolve anything – that was beyond their capacity – their duty was to ensure her safety, as far as they were able.

Provided by John Blackler

CASE STUDY 11.4

Beverly is a new social worker in a residential facility for elderly people in a rural area. There are few jobs for social workers in the area, and high unemployment generally. At the hostel, strict rules apply. Husbands and wives live in different wards and are only allowed to meet on an open veranda under supervision.

During her first month at the hostel, Beverly is approached by a resident asking for assistance to have the rules changed. He says that it is ridiculous to pay so much money to live in something like a gaol, but he has no choice as he cannot care for his wife alone and there are no other residential services in the area. Beverly knows that the last social worker was dismissed for being a troublemaker.

Provided by Wendy Bowles

CASE STUDY 11.5

Elizabeth Johnson, a community social worker on a disability team has been asked to visit a couple who want help to apply for a Department of Housing home. The husband Trevor is recovering from a motorbike accident which left him with head injuries and severe pain from other injuries. He met his wife Julie at the rehabilitation centre. Julie was also in a motorbike accident in which she lost her foot. Trevor and Julie have a new baby and an 18-month-old baby.

When Elizabeth visits the couple in their small, rented, one bedroom apartment, she notices what a mess the place is in. Soiled nappies are piled in a corner of the kitchen, half filled babies' bottles lie about on the kitchen bench with other dirty washing up and overflowing ashtrays, and the 18-month-old is playing with the cat food dish on the floor. Elizabeth notices a smoky smell which is not tobacco.

Trevor and Julie welcome Elizabeth enthusiastically, saying what a help the last social worker from the disability team was. They also say they are glad that Elizabeth does not work for 'the welfare' because they have been having trouble with neighbours lately who keep reporting them for the noise that comes from their flat. They say that one neighbour in particular 'is trying to get our babies taken away'. That is why they are applying for a Department of Housing home, so that they can get away from the neighbours and have some peace, as well as extra space. Julie explains that the apartment is messy because 'we are all crammed in one bedroom here and there isn't room to swing the cat'.

Both Julie and Trevor have bruises on their faces and arms. When Elizabeth enquires if there has been an accident, they say that they have been 'stressed out' lately and that sometimes their fights get out of hand. The toddler on the floor does not seem to be bruised. The baby is nowhere in sight. Elizabeth helps Trevor and Julie fill in the application form for the Department of Housing.

As she leaves Trevor and Julie ask her to come back soon. 'The last social worker was such a help. The neighbours will stay off our backs if someone comes to see us regularly. People from your place are much better than the welfare. Maybe you can get us some more help with Trevor's pain levels too.'

Provided by Wendy Bowles

CASE STUDY 11.6

Dorothy is an elderly widow who lives in her own home. She receives some assistance in daily living from Home Care, and Meals on Wheels calls twice each week. She is reasonably active and mentally alert but has few friends. Most of her social contact is provided by her married daughter who lives nearby. Recently, Home Care staff have noticed that she seems depressed. She does not seem to be taking as much care with her personal hygiene and is losing weight. She told the workers that her daughter never came to visit her any more and she asked them to tell her daughter to come and visit. When the daughter was contacted, she told the Home Care Branch Manager that her mother was far too demanding and she was 'going to teach her' that she had her own life to lead.

Mike Collingridge and Seumas Miller (1997) 'Filial responsibility and the care of the aged', Journal of Applied Philosophy

CASE STUDY 11.7

The onset of sexual activity was examined with respect to the decade in which people were born. Half the men born between 1941 and 1950 had vaginal intercourse by age 18 and this declined to 16 for men born between 1981 and 1986. For women the age at first vaginal intercourse declined from 19 to 16. Contraceptive use at first intercourse increased from less than 30% of men and women in the 1950s to over 90% in the 2000s. The age at first experience of oral sex declined even more steeply over that period and now typically occurs around the time of first vaginal intercourse rather than some years afterward. The age of first homosexual experience was higher than the age of first heterosexual experience. Thus, the majority of young people in the final years of school today will have commenced sexual activity, and this highlights the importance of sex education in schools.

Heterosexual men reported more partners over their lifetime, in the last five years and in the last year than did heterosexual women, with 15.1% of heterosexual men and 8.5% of heterosexual women reporting multiple sexual partners in the last year, although these partnerships were not necessarily concurrent. People who identified as homosexual or bisexual reported more partners than did those who identified as heterosexual. Homosexual men and bisexual men and women had had more partners than lesbians.

One person in four had not had sex in the previous four weeks and most people in the survey, both men and women, wanted more sex than they were having. Most people had sex less than twice a week, whereas 23.4% of men and 8.3% of women would like to have had sex daily or more often. Those who had been in heterosexual relationships for at least twelve months had sex on average 1.84 times a week in the last four weeks, with younger people having sex more frequently.

Most people in heterosexual relationships found sex very or extremely pleasurable (90.3% men and 79.1% women) with high levels of emotional satisfaction also reported (87.5% men and 79.1% women). Physical pleasure in sex was strongly related to emotional satisfaction.

Over three quarters of men and women agreed that premarital sex is acceptable. There was little difference between men and women. Three quarters of respondents agreed that oral sex is sex, again with no gender differences, and three quarters also agreed that having an affair outside a committed relationship is wrong. The majority agreed that having sex is important to wellbeing.

In this study 97.4% of men identified as heterosexual, 1.6% as gay and 0.9% as bisexual. For women 97.7% identified as heterosexual, 0.8% as gay and 1.4% as bisexual. Nevertheless, 8.6% of men and 15.1% of women reported either feelings of attraction to the same sex or some sexual experience with the same sex. Half the men and two thirds of the women who had same sex sexual experience regarded themselves as heterosexual rather than homosexual. This illustrates that same sex attraction and experience are more common in Australia than is indicated by the relatively few people reporting a homosexual or bisexual identity.

Australian Research Centre in Sex, Health and Society (2003)
Sex in Australia: Summary Findings of the Australian Study of Health and Relationships

CASE STUDY 11.8

She ask me, How was it with your children daddy?

The girls had a little separate room, I say, off to itself, connected to the house by a little plank walk. Nobody ever come in there but Mama. But one time when mama not at home, he come. Told me he want me to trim his hair. He bring the scissors and comb and brush and a stool. While I trim his hair he look at me funny. He a little nervous too, but I don't know why, til he grab hold of me and cram me up tween his legs.

I lay there quiet listening to Shug breathe.

It hurt me, you know, I say. I was going on fourteen. I never even thought bout men having nothing down there so big. It scare me just to see it. And the way it poke itself and grow.

Shug so quiet I think she sleep.

After he through, I say, he make me finish trimming his hair.

I sneak a look at Shug.

Oh, Miss Celie, she say. And put her arms around me. They black and smooth and sort of glowy from the lamplight.

I start to cry too. I cry and cry and cry. Seem like it all come back to me, laying there in Shug arms. How it hurt and how much I was surprise. How it stung while I finish trimming his hair. How the blood drip down my leg and mess up my stocking. How he never look at me straight after that …

She say, I love you, Miss Celie. And then she haul off and kiss me on the mouth.

Um, she say, like she surprise. I kiss her back, say, *um,* too. Us kiss and kiss til us can't hardly kiss no more. Then us touch each other.

I don't know nothing bout it, I say to Shug.

I don't know much, she say.

Then I feels something real soft and wet on my breast, feel like one of my little lost babies mouth.

Way after while, I act like a little lost baby too.

Alice Walker (1982) The Color Purple

CASE STUDY 11.9

I like tying up my lover and she likes it too. I will not be made to feel guilty as if I am doing something violative. I was that good girl, that obedient child. Feminism said let go. You can do what a man does. I like tying her wrists to the bed, I like gagging her, I like dripping hot wax on her breasts. It is not the same as when a man does it. She and I are equals, the same. There is no moral atrocity or political big deal … I have more in common with the so-called rapist, the knowing so-called rapist, the one who seduces, at least a little, and uses force because it's sexy; it is sexy; I like doing it and the men I know know I like doing it, to a woman; they are pro-gay. I'm an ally and I will get tenure. The so-called rapists in my university are educated men. We like sex and to each his own … I have been hurt but it was a long time ago. I'm not the same girl.

Andrea Dworkin (1991) Mercy

CASE STUDY 11.10

Never before or since have five column inches on an inside page generated such fury from our readers.

The story began routinely enough. A 25-year-old man from a

nearby town was found hanging from a tree in his backyard.

The *Free Press* (Mankato, MN) ran a short story about the death with few details, noting only that it was being investigated. Sheriff's deputies were unusually tight-lipped about the case. In the week following the initial story, rumour fed upon speculation until several bizarre murder theories had circulated.

Interest in the death was heightened because the young man was a well-known teacher of the physically and mentally disabled. A local lecturer and volunteer, he was admired by many.

A week after a neighbour had found the nude body, the sheriff's department and coroner released a ruling on the death: accidental, due to sexual asphyxia.

Even among our well-read news staff, few knew much about sexual asphyxiation. The practice, also called autoerotic asphyxiation, involves attempting to reach a heightened sexual orgasm by cutting off the oxygen and blood supply to the head during masturbation. Not everyone who tries it dies, but accidental death often occurs when the person loses consciousness and falls forward, being strangled by the rope or belt tied to his neck.

The question came immediately to mind: If we were somewhat shocked would our readers be at all prepared? The answer, we knew, was an unequivocal 'no.'

Editors, the reporter and the publisher met to discuss the options. The rumors were too widespread to even consider letting the incident pass without mention. Could we say the death was definitely not foul play and leave it at that? It would, of course, leave readers with the impression that it was a suicide – a normally unsettling cause of death for family and friends to accept, but in this case a less embarrassing conclusion than the true circumstances.

The argument to simply rule out foul play was buttressed by the fact that radio and television stations did not give the official cause of death in their reports immediately following the ruling.

But other reporters and editors argued that the death involved a week-long sheriff's investigation and had gained wide public interest. A hazy article would not adequately answer all the questions.

And what about the newspaper's role as an educator to others who may have thought about experimenting with the potentially deadly practice?

'Doc' Sanford, the savvy, progressive coroner who ruled on the death, came to the newspaper office arguing for publication of full details. 'This is being done by a lot of people out there. It's dangerous and they should know it', he said.

After some quick studying we learned that accidental death from the practice, is indeed, no fluke. According to an FBI study an estimated 500–1000 people die yearly in the US from sexual asphyxiation. The agency describes most victims as male adolescents or young adults who are happy and well-adjusted. Besides the deaths, many people are brain damaged by the practice ...

After examining all the arguments, we went ahead with an article we hoped would fulfil our public record reporting obligations, warn others about a dangerous practice, and at the same time, not give undue attention to the story. A short, five-inch story on the bottom of page 15 gave the coroner's ruling of the death with a brief, clinical description of sexual asphyxia.

We expected criticism. But no-one was prepared for the onslaught of outrage. Telephone calls and letters to the editor continued for weeks.

From the mother: 'One word – accidental – would have explained it all. [The story] didn't serve any good purpose, but only angered and hurt people.'

From a minister: '... Your article, written from the very depth of the sewer, was totally uncalled for.'

Even many staff members' families and friends thought the newspaper was far out of bounds.

A couple of years later, we still are angrily confronted about 'that story.'

Would we have done the story the same way knowing the outcome?

Tim Krohn (1990) 'Deadly lesson: Warning about sexual asphyxiation – A respected teacher dies while performing a dangerous sex act. How do you warn others when readers don't want to hear it?'

ETHICAL ANALYSIS

Institution of the family

When we talk of a family this can mean two things (Alexandra, Matthews, and Miller 2002):

1) *Biological family.* First, we may be speaking in biological terms. In this sense people of the same blood – parents and children for example – are members of the same family. Whether people are or are not members of a family in this sense is a matter of brute fact; it is independent of our perceptions and beliefs. Thus, it would be quite possible for someone to meet a person of his or her own (biological) family and not realise it.

2) *Social family.* Second, we may be speaking in social terms. If so, whether some group of people count as a family is a matter of social conventions. Here perceptions and beliefs are of primary importance. Though most of us, most of the time, have little hesitation deciding whether some people are family in this social sense, it is more difficult to provide a watertight definition of this kind of family.

In the past, in societies like Australia, there tended to be a strong, though not invariable, correlation between the biological and social senses of the term 'family'. This was brought about by the acceptance of the norms of exclusive, lifelong heterosexual marriage. This meant that members of a biological family tended to live together as a social family. (You should note here, incidentally, that when we talk about norms we are referring to standards of behaviour that people have accepted. We are not necessarily advocating that these standards should be accepted.) The changes to these norms have meant that more groups that are not defined as biological families are likely to be recognised as families in the social sense. The Australian Bureau of Statistics (ABS) captures the broadness of the current understanding of social families in its definition of a family as:

> Two or more persons, one of whom is aged
> 15 years and over, who are related by blood,
> marriage (registered or de facto), adoption, step or
> fostering; and who are usually resident in the same
> household. The basis of a family is formed by
> identifying the presence of a couple relationship,
> lone parent–child relationship or other blood
> relationship (ABS 2000).

This definition allows for a wide range of combinations of people to count as a family, including childless homosexual couples, single mothers living with their children, grandparents living with grandchildren, as well as the so-called 'nuclear family' of married mother, father and child or children. (See case studies 11.1 and 11.4 as well as 11.2, 11.3 and 11.5.) The changes of norms both reflect and contribute to the greater diversity in family arrangements. For example, the ABS measured almost 300 percent growth in the number of single parent families just in the 30 years between 1971 and 2001. An important figure relates to the way younger adults these days are delaying marriage, and presumably there will be some correlation between such rates and having children. According to the ABS:

> By the time the group of people born in 1965–69
> had reached 30–34 years, nearly 24% remained
> unmarried, almost twice as many as those born
> 15 years earlier, when 13% remained unmarried at
> the same age. (ABS 2002)

The trends in family composition reflect a number of factors. A very important one is Australia's ageing population. In 1901, 4 percent of the population were 65 or over; in 2001, the figure was 12 percent; it is projected to go to 18 percent by 2020. This has implications for the obligations children have to their ageing parents, so-called filial responsibilities. (See case study 11.6.) We discuss these obligations further below.

The next 20 years are likely to see changes in family composition. It is thought that childless couples will become the most common type of family. (See case study 11.4.) ABS projections are that by around 2020 they will constitute 42 percent of all families. This tendency will be caused partly by the increase in the ageing population, but also because couples are choosing not to have children. The roles of women are changing because they are choosing to participate in work and education, and so delaying pregnancy. Thus, it is projected that although the absolute numbers of couple families with children will remain static until 2020, relative to overall numbers of families they will decline from 49 percent to 40 percent. An additional factor in the composition of families is the increase in rates of divorce. By 2020 it is thought there will be about 1.1 million single-parent family structures (up from 742 000 in 1996). Again, there are implications for the role-responsibilities within these new family arrangements. Older siblings, for example, will tend to bear the responsibility for looking after younger family members.

The norms regarding what counts as a family have been changing. But so too have the kinds of behaviour thought proper to the various roles within the family. The norms regulating the relation of husbands to their wives, and fathers to their children have relaxed considerably over the past couple of decades. The place of women is no longer automatically seen as 'in the home', as the figures above would indicate.

The family, understood in this broad way, is a thriving institution in Australian society. Almost everyone in Australia grows up in a family, and most people establish families of their own in their adult lives. According to the ABS, over 80 percent of Australians live in household families. Of those who do not, a number are obviously in the transitional stage between leaving their childhood family and beginning a family of their own, so will sooner or later return to family living, while an increasing number are old people who have been left alone by the death of a partner. Case study 11.6 reveals some of the problems that this creates, both in terms of physical care and loneliness. In other words, most people in Australia live most of their lives in a family setting.

The family is an important institution in a number of ways. First, it plays a fundamental role in the socialisation of children. It is where they learn how to speak a language, how to eat, establish a sexual identity, learn what the conventions and customs of the society are, and so on. Consider here the problems posed when parents are unable to exercise authority in relation to their children and, therefore, the impact on the process of education/socialisation. (See case study 11.2.) Second, and relatedly, it is the most important site of the moralisation of children. It is where they learn right from wrong, concern for others rather than mere childish selfishness, to take responsibility for their actions, and so on. Consider the problems generated by negligent parenting (see case study 11.5) or by parents who harm their children by, for example, sexually abusing them (see case study 11.8). Third, the family is of great importance in the economic life of the community. Much of the (mainly unpaid) labour of modern life occurs within the family home, in the form of cooking, cleaning, gardening, and so on. Most of the spending of individuals is on goods and services that are consumed by family members within the home; the family home itself is the most significant purchase that most people make. Finally, since family members spend so much time with each other, the quality of individuals' private lives is largely determined by the nature of their interaction with fellow family members. At its best, family life can provide a haven from the stresses of the workaday world, and is marked by reciprocal affection and consideration; at its worst it is marked by violence, exploitation and hatred. (See case study 11.3.)

In recent years the more extreme forms of family dysfunction, such as child abuse and domestic violence, have received a good deal of publicity. (See case studies 11.8 and 11.3, respectively.) By its very nature, much of this activity is concealed. It usually takes place away from outsiders, and often the victims are too ashamed, frightened, or dependent on the perpetrators – and in the case of young children, too inarticulate – to report it. It is therefore difficult to get an accurate picture of how much actually goes on. Reported child abuse in recent years has risen, for example, but it is possible that this rise is due more to changes in reporting procedures – teachers and doctors are now required to report suspected child abuse – and attitudes, than it is to an actual rise in child abuse itself. It is worth noting that certain forms of behaviour previously thought to be acceptable or at least something to be 'kept in the family' are now seen as intolerable. For instance, physical violence against children in the form of slapping, hitting or even beating and whipping in the name of discipline were normal in many families until quite recently, and only in the last few decades have the Australian states enacted legislation against rape in marriage.

Despite the difficulties inherent in getting a clear picture of domestic violence and the like, some reliable figures do indicate the extent of the problem. Figures on homicides, for instance, tend to be very reliable, for obvious reasons. About 40 percent of all homicides in Australia take place within the family (as against 11 percent between people who do not know each other). Of those, roughly a third involve parents and children, and half involve spouses.

Given the importance of the family, it is inevitable that the government or state will take an interest in it. The relationship between family and the state is complex, and continually being renegotiated. The tendency, however, is for the state to be more intrusive in family matters. We see this tendency at work, for instance, in its increasing involvement in relation to domestic violence and child abuse. Going further back, attendance at school only became compulsory in the 19th century, removing the choice as to whether children would receive an education from the family circle.

Love, sex and the family

Accompanying changes in family life have been changes in norms governing sexual behaviour. (See case study 11.7 for a snapshot.) Just as there is ongoing controversy and disagreement about the desirability of the changes in the norms of family life, so too are the norms covering sexual behaviour debated. (See case study 11.9.) To begin with we will describe some standard norms of sexual morality, particularly as they apply to family life, then consider whether there is any systematic way of making judgments about sexual morality.

Traditional sexual morality is the code which was generally accepted until relatively recently in countries like Australia, and is still accepted by a significant number of people. To say that this code was accepted does not of course mean that people always acted according to it. In many cases they may have only paid it lip service. Nevertheless, most people would have claimed to have accepted it, and would have tried to conceal any deviations from it. It is marked by the following features:

- Sexual relations should occur: (a) only between people who are married to each other (marriage fidelity), (b) only between people of opposite sexes (heterosexuality), and (c) never before marriage (premarital chastity).
- Ideally marriage should be romantically based (romantic attraction is the proper foundation for the choice of marriage partner).
- Child rearing should take place within marriage.
- Marriage should be permanent (there should be a strong commitment to the maintenance of a marriage by both parties).
- Marriage is for procreation: children should issue from it. (This was not accepted by all who agreed with the other demands of traditional morality.)

Correspondingly of course, traditionalists think there are a number of sexual vices such as premarital sex, bearing of illegitimate children, marital infidelity, lack of commitment to the marriage and so on. The traditional model is taken to be absolutist, or very nearly absolutist, about ruling out such vices, that is, it holds that engaging in them can never, or almost never, be justified (the prohibition on them is 'absolute') (Finnis 1980). It may be this absolutism that, in the face of a variety of external cultural changes, has brought about the downfall of the traditional approach to these matters.

Though some people still espouse traditional sexual morality, it is now not the only system of sexual morality enjoying much support, and indeed much evidence suggests that it is on the wane. Marriage is no longer the only acceptable setting for sexual relations, or for raising children. Many people now accept (at least in the sense of living according to) what might be called conventional sexual morality. It is marked by the following features:

- Romantically-based sex: romantic attraction is the proper basis for sexual relationships between two people.
- Fidelity/exclusivity: a person restricts their sexual relationships to one person at a time.
- Joint procreative responsibility: men and women share responsibility for procreation and the raising of children.
- Child rearing within a committed relationship: children are best raised by adults who are themselves involved in a committed relationship.

Again a number of corresponding sexual vices, such as infidelity, irresponsibility towards children and so on also exist.

This form of sexual morality differs from traditional sexual morality in some respects. One of the important differences is that there is no requirement that sex should be heterosexual. (See case study 11.9.) This does not amount to a positive endorsement of homosexuality. There are four kinds of moral attitudes one can take towards behaviour:

1) approval, where it is seen as good and to be encouraged;
2) disapproval, where it is seen as bad, and to be stopped if possible;
3) indifference, where it is seen as neither good nor bad; and
4) tolerance.

To adopt an attitude of tolerance towards an activity is to disapprove it while stopping short of its prevention. Many of those who accept conventional morality may tolerate homosexuality, but they would disapprove of, say, polygamous arrangements. Conventional morality places less stress than traditional morality on the importance of the family. It allows, for instance that people who do not live together and form a family may legitimately be in a sexual relationship with each other.

In other ways conventional morality is like traditional morality. For example, given its insistence that romantic attraction is the basis of the choice of a marriage partner, and that sex should occur only between married people, traditional morality would seem to agree with conventional morality that sex should be romantically based. Sufficient overlap does in fact exist between these two codes for some people to accept elements of both, or move from one to the other without too much strain. So, some people are quite happy to accept that people should have a free choice of sexual partners until they have children, at which point they should marry and accept the restrictions of traditional morality.

Some people have denied that there is any specifically sexual morality (Primoratz 1999). This approach is summed up in the claim that 'having sex with someone is no more important than having dinner with them'. This is not to say that in sexual matters anything goes, any more than it does at the dining table. No doubt we should not force others to dine with us at gun point, and even if they dine with us voluntarily we should not try to foist our taste in food on them, not act in ways which will detract from their enjoyment of the occasion, and so on. Similarly (it almost goes without saying) no-one should force another to have sex against his or her will, nor should the needs of others be ignored and so on. These are moral requirements, but they are applications of moral requirements of a general nature, which can be applied to a whole range of situations, rather than requirements of a specifically sexual morality. So, those who reject any kind of sexual morality, are of course still bound by morality as it applies to behaviour generally. But they deny that there are any special norms associated with sexual activity as claimed by the traditionalists and the conventionalists.

If one accepts that there is no special sexual morality, some of the controversial issues about it and the family come to seem like non-issues. If having sex with someone is no more significant in itself than sharing dinner, then presumably there is no virtue in having sex only with marriage partners, or with only one person for periods of time, indeed nothing wrong with having sex with lots of people at the same time, regardless of their gender. (Again, this is not to say anything goes since one is still bound by morality generally. There are strong moral arguments for thinking that sexual activity should, for example, occur only between consenting adults.)

Proponents of the 'no sexual morality' theory would see no relation between sexual morality and family life. They may or may not support family life, but even if they did there could be no question that sexual relationships must be confined to one's companion in that life.

One way of deciding between the accounts is to think about the various functions sexual activity plays. One obvious function for sex is that it brings pleasure. Usually, after all, it is the desire for pleasure that motivates people to engage in sexual activity. If we considered that the only function of sex is to bring pleasure, then this would seem to support the 'no distinctive sexual morality' theory. After all, in itself pleasure is a good thing and normally we think that people should be allowed to engage in pleasurable pursuits (playing golf, riding the roller coaster, etc) provided they do not hurt others in the process or ignore more important claims on their time.

In general, there is no doubt that sex fulfils a pleasure-seeking function. But of course this can be more or less fulfilled regardless of which model of sexual morality we adopt. Moreover, pleasure is clearly not the only function of sex. In order to see this consider again the analogy with eating. People take pleasure in eating, just as they do with sex, and eating satisfies a physical appetite, just as sex does. But it would be wrong to say that gaining pleasure is the sole function of eating, or even the main function. For eating plays a role in our physical being; it provides life-giving nourishment. If we suddenly ceased to gain pleasure from eating, we would nonetheless continue to perform that activity to stay alive. Indeed, one could say that the gaining of pleasure, rather than being the only purpose of eating, provides a stimulus or prompt which helps us achieve the end of gaining nourishment. One could even say that allowing the pleasurable aspects of eating to become an end in itself would be a very bad thing, a kind of perversion, leading to gluttony and ill-health. Similar things can be said about sex. In the right circumstances sexual activity is obviously pleasurable, but this should not be seen as its sole end, and indeed arguably the pleasure of sex could be regarded as the stimulus for sexual activity that fulfils other ends. Certainly regarding pleasure as the only function of sex can lead to an analogous form of gluttony.

Besides pleasure, then, what are the ends of sexual activity? The answer is usually one or both of the following:

- Unification: the point of sex is to bind sexual partners together in a relationship of special intimacy, love and trust.
- Procreation: the point of sex is to produce offspring.

If both these claims are accepted, they would seem to support traditional morality, which emphasises the special nature of sexual union and its role in procreation. Acceptance of the first claim alone, that the point of sex is to bind sexual partners together, would seem to support conventional sexual morality, which also emphasises the special nature of sexual union, but denies that this must be accompanied by procreation. Consider the ageing couple in case study 11.4 who are being denied the possibility of sexual union in the context of an aged care facility.

Should we accept either of these claims regarding the end(s) of sex? If we do we would also seem to accept that sex which is not aimed at achieving these ends will count as perverse, just as eating without hunger is considered gluttony. In trying to discover the purpose or end of some activity, we need to be careful not to confuse frequent or typical outcomes of that activity with its purpose. Having a sore stomach may be the result of uncontrolled laughter, but this hardly shows that the good which is aimed at by laughing is the production of sore stomachs. Similarly, though procreation may be the frequent (though obviously not invariable) outcome of sexual intercourse, that hardly demonstrates that procreation is the good end or purpose of sexual intercourse. While in the case of eating we know that lack of nourishment is bad for the individual, failure to procreate need not be bad for the individual. Rather, in some cases procreation itself is bad for the individual; pregnancy may be the last thing a woman needs if she is sick or living in poverty for example. Moreover, if all those who engage in sexual activity invariably procreate, then procreation may be bad for us collectively, given the problems we face of overpopulation.

Again, though unification may often accompany sexual activity, there are problems in thinking that it must be (one of) its ends. If we accept this claim, for instance, it seems that two people who come together purely for the sake of giving and receiving pleasure and then go their separate ways with no thought of meeting again will be counted as acting perversely. And what about people who, for one reason or another, are unable to form lasting attachments with sexual partners? Must they therefore be denied a sexual life?

Summing up, what this analysis has shown is that sexual activity can fulfil three separate functions: the provision of pleasure, unification and procreation. In deciding which of the theories of sexual morality we should adopt we emphasised that we should focus on the desirable functions of the activity. Pleasure is a desirable part of sexual activity, but it alone cannot be regarded as *the* function of sex. Procreation is desirable too, but again we cannot regard it as singularly important. If sex never led to procreation, the human race would cease to exist. If sex always led to procreation we might also cease to exist, although for other reasons! Unification is desirable, but if we regard it as central to sexual activity, then we implausibly rule out the possibility of a sexual life for those who reject the forming of partnerships.

If we accept the claim that sexual activity can have these three functions, with value attached to each function, this allows us to draw some conclusions regarding which theory of sexual morality is to be preferred. The analysis points to a pluralist approach. The pluralist in this context says that we ought to approve of a variety of sexual norms, and that individuals who engage in the range of practices approved are to be respected, or at worst, tolerated. The upshot is that the conventional model of sexual morality comes out the best. The 'no distinctive sexual morality' position omits too much of what we think are the desirable aspects of sex; the traditional view is too restrictive in what it permits.

Ethics of vulnerability: filial responsibility

Governments of Western economies are currently wrestling with burgeoning social welfare bills associated with their demographically ageing populations. This makes filial responsibility (the duty of children to take care of their parents) an issue of great concern (Collingridge and Miller 1997). A family responsibility policy might, for example, require adult children, if they were not in a position to physically care for their aged parents, to contribute to the costs of nursing home care in circumstances where parents could not do so themselves. But why stop there? There seems no logical reason (but there may be moral and political reasons) why a filial responsibility policy should only be seen as a way of reducing pressure on the health and welfare budget.

Both public policy (reflected in the law) and conventional ethics assumes a duty of care to children by their parents. We have laws to protect children when the appropriate level of care is not provided. Similarly, both law and morality accept the notion of obligation between spouses, although the legal and moral imperatives are probably less strong now than they were in the past. Still, there is no doubt that these obligations exist. It is harder, however, to provide a ground or justification for such special obligations. It is even more difficult to find a justification for these obligations when the boundary encompassing those coming within the special family relationship expands. Thus, it is generally taken as axiomatic that parents are 'entitled to be given honour, reverence and filial affection' from their adult children. However, to suggest that adult children have wider moral responsibilities towards their aged parents, including in particular, material assistance, is rather more problematic. To translate such moral responsibilities into public policies is equally fraught.

The issue of filial responsibility, while not explicitly referred to as such has, however, arisen recently in a different form, namely in relation to the abuse and neglect of the elderly. The NSW Task Force on Abuse of Older People (1992) defined neglect as:

> The failure to provide adequate food, shelter,
> clothing or dental care. This may involve
> the refusal to permit other people to provide
> appropriate care. Examples include abandonment,
> non provision of nourishing food, adequate
> clothing or shelter, inappropriate use of
> medication (including over-medication) and poor
> hygiene or personal care.

This 'taken for granted' definition (which we might add is common in the literature on abuse of the elderly) is based on an assumption that someone (spouse, adult child, other family member, third party) has not only taken on the responsibility for care, but has also failed to adequately discharge that responsibility. Given that under Australian law there is no general obligation for adult children to care for their parents, or indeed for any relative (other than spouses and under-age children), unless there is some other relationship between adult child and parent, such as a contractual or quasi-contractual relationship, the notion of responsibility to care is severely stretched.

The problem of moral, if not legal culpability, is further stretched in the case of psychological abuse. This is defined as the infliction of mental anguish, including actions that lead to fear of violence, to isolation, or deprivation, feelings of shame, indignity or powerlessness.

Consider case study 11.6. According to some definitions of elder abuse the daughter is 'psychologically abusing' her mother, causing physical harm as a consequence of the mother's self-neglect. Leaving aside for the moment the question of whether there are grounds for intervention to 'protect Dorothy from harm', are we able to say that the daughter is morally culpable in some way? Does she have an obligation to visit? Can the obligation be enforced? If the daughter is morally culpable, what is the underlying basis of her obligation which she has failed to live up to? On a more practical note, what can health or welfare services possibly have to offer a woman who is literally making herself sick through grief except, perhaps, psychiatric services?

Much of the research both here and overseas shows that care of defined sections of the community has always been a shared responsibility between the state and the family. A large part of that burden has been borne by the state. So what is the current relationship between care of the aged by families and public provision? Given that there was never a high level of family responsibility, what evidence suggests that family responsibility has deteriorated or that families are, in some way, shirking their moral and social responsibilities?

The research on the aged in Australia and overseas also reveals the importance of autonomy in the lives of the elderly. A substantial section of the aged live alone, usually by choice. Even where they need assistance in some aspect of daily living, research suggests many would prefer not to rely on family or kinship networks, and choose instead to seek formal social service support. Nevertheless, as research has shown, adult children tend to regard the support of their parents or grandparents as a matter of obligation, but there is only qualified acceptance by the aged themselves of help that cannot be reciprocated. Crucially the elderly have a firm belief in their right to government services. They see these as an accepted method of avoiding being a burden on their family.

The idea that adult children have a strong sense of obligation is supported by research from Canada (Wolfson et al 1993). This research identified a difference between what children thought they should do and what they could do for their parents. Emotional support was the one thing most families could provide. This seems to confirm the view that the type of support that is important for the wellbeing of elderly people is expressive support, which may be offered by kin, but can also be provided by a wider network of friends.

THREE THEORIES OF FILIAL RESPONSIBILITY

So, do children have responsibilities to care for their aged parents? To help determine whether they do, and the extent to which these responsibilities exist, we will consider the three most influential models of filial responsibility. These are the Reciprocity model, the Needs-based model and the Friendship model.

Reciprocity model

According to the Reciprocity model of filial responsibility, adult children have duties to care for their aged parents because their parents brought them into existence, nurtured them, educated them and provided them with material benefits, including food, clothing and shelter (Jecker 1989). Presumably, on this view, the kind and extent of benefits provided by parents determines the kind and extent of the obligations owed by adult children to their parents.

The Reciprocity model confronts a number of objections. In relation to the alleged reciprocal obligation based on biological parenthood, consider two people who have a child because they are paid to do so by some third party who wants a child. First, what exactly is owed by such a child to his parents? What is an appropriate 'repayment' to a person who brought someone into existence for money, but is otherwise an uncaring stranger? Second, is being brought into existence a benefit? Granted it is certainly a necessary condition for being able to receive benefits. Moreover, your parents were not the only ones to provide a necessary link for your existence; after all, your grandparents provided such a link, and their parents, and so on, all the way back through the generations.

In relation to the alleged reciprocal obligations based on provision of material benefits, the actual needs of aged parents – according to the Reciprocity model – make no difference to what they are owed by their adult children. If a particular parent provided a child with an abundance of material benefits, then, on the Reciprocity model, this child owes that parent a corresponding abundance of material goods, notwithstanding the fact that his parent is extremely wealthy and in no need of material support. Conversely the (perhaps very rich) offspring of a poor parent owes her parent very little in material support, since she received very little. These consequences of the Reciprocity model conflict with what we intuitively take the filial obligations in such cases to be.

Finally, in relation to the benefits of love and affection provided by parents to their children, the Reciprocity model is also inadequate. Relationships of love and affection cannot be understood simply in terms of reciprocal obligations. A child who loves his parents would normally try to assist them at least in part out of love, rather than because he felt he owed them for loving him.

The apparent inadequacy of the Reciprocity model, with its emphasis on what the parent has done for the child, suggests a needs-based account. Adult children ought to assist their parents because their parents need to be helped.

Needs-based model

According to the Needs-based model adult children should provide their elderly parents with material and other forms of assistance because their parents need such assistance, and need is a fundamental moral consideration (Goodin 1985). One strength of this model is that it explains why adult children with rich elderly parents do not have an obligation to provide material benefits to their parents, while adult children with destitute elderly parents, do have such an obligation. Further, this view does not imply that one might have obligations to a person simply because that person is one's biological parent. So, on this approach, if your biological father was a sperm donor, but nothing more, you do not have obligations towards him simply in virtue of that fact.

Unfortunately, though, the Needs-based model fails to adequately distinguish filial obligations from other obligations where the needs of an individual are in play. Let us grant that there are obligations to satisfy the needs of aged parents. Why are adult children the ones obligated? The existence of objective needs may generate obligations on someone or other to satisfy those needs, but not adult children in particular. Perhaps those who are best able to satisfy the given needs of particular elderly parents are, as a matter of contingent fact, their adult children. But this is not necessarily the case. Certainly in relation to material needs the state is often the best able to assist the aged. And in relation to psychological needs, persons other than adult children may be better able to assist because they are trained or because they are more compatible in terms of personality, life history or whatever.

A further problem with the Needs-based model is that like the

Reciprocity model, it fails to accommodate the emotional attitudes that characterise parent–child relationships. Clearly, adult children are often motivated to care for their parents by feelings of love and affection.

Friendship model
According to this model (English 1979), children owe nothing to their parents, since they did not consent either to being brought into the world, or to receiving the benefits provided by their parents. Moreover, they have no special duties to parents in their old age other than the general duty to help those in need. However in so far as children, and adult children in particular, have a friendship-like relationship with their parents, they ought to assist them in the ways friends would normally help one another. However such assistance would be given out of love as opposed to duty, since acting for the sake of duty is – according to this model – inconsistent with friendship.

There are several objections to the Friendship model. First, the assertion that adult children are not duty-bound to their parents is a claim that needs to be substantiated. Even if (in some cases) children do have a relation to their parents a bit like a friendship, the parent–child relation does not dissolve as well. So, the duties this relationship creates may remain. Or at least it has to be shown that they do not. Second, it is highly debatable that one can have a parent as a friend in the proper sense of that term. Although some overlap exists between the idea of a friendship and a parent–child relationship – mutual affection, the desire for shared experiences, the disposition to benefit and promote the interests of the other – there is a great deal of difference as well. For example, friends, to some extent, choose one another, stand as equals in a relationship, and have a much greater independence in the relationship than is the case with parents and their children. Finally, and most damagingly to this model, if our parents were no more than very close friends, then the termination conditions which apply to friendships would also apply to parent–child relations. That one's relationship with parents could end as easily as one's relationship with a friend is just a little hard to swallow.

Readings

Alexandra, Andrew, Matthews, Steve and Miller, Seumas (2002) *Reasons, Values and Institutions*, Tertiary Press, Croydon.

Australian Bureau of Statistics (2000) 'Labour force status and other characteristics of families, Australia', ABS Cat no 6224.0.

— (2002) 'Australian social trends 2002, Family-living arrangements: Changes across Australian generations', ABS Cat no 4102.0.

Australian Research Centre in Sex, Health and Society, *Sex in Australia: Summary Findings of the Australian Study of Health and Relationships* (2003) La Trobe University, available at <http://www.latrobe.edu.au/ashr/> (accessed 23/1/09).

Collingridge, Michael and Miller, Seumas (1997) 'Filial responsibility and the care of the aged', *Journal of Applied Philosophy*, vol 14, no 2, p 123.

Dworkin, Andrea (1991) *Mercy*, Four Walls Eight Windows, New York, pp 341–42.

English, Jane (1979) 'What do grown children owe their parents' in O'Neill, Onora (ed) *Having Children*, Oxford University Press, New York.

Finnis, John (1980) *Natural Law and Natural Rights*, Oxford University Press, Oxford.

Goodin, Robert (1985) *Protecting the Vulnerable*, University of Chicago Press, Chicago.

Hoff Sommers, Christina (1986) 'Filial morality', *Journal of Philosophy*, vol 83, no 8, pp 439–56.

Jecker, Nancy (1989) 'Are filial duties unfounded?', *American Philosophical Quarterly*, vol 26, no 1, pp 73–80.

Keller, Simon (2006) 'Four theories of filial duty', *Philosophical Quarterly*, vol 56, no 223, pp 254–74.

Krohn, Tim (1990) 'Deadly lesson: Warning about sexual asphyxiation – A respected teacher dies while performing a dangerous sex act. How do you warn others when readers don't want to hear it?', *FineLine: The Newsletter on Journalism Ethics*, vol 2, no 2 (May), p 4, available at <http://journalism.indiana.edu/resources/ethics/sensitive-news-topics/deadly-lesson> (accessed 23/1/09).

Moller Okin, Susan (1987) *Justice, Gender and the Family*, Basic Books, New York.

New South Wales Task Force on Abuse of Older People (1992) *Abuse of Older People in their Homes*, Office on Ageing, Sydney.

Primoratz, Igor (1999) *Ethics and Sex*, Routledge, London.

Walker, Alice (1982) *The Color Purple*, Washington Square Press, New York, pp 108–09.

Wolfson, Christina, Handfield-Jones, Richard, Glass, Kathleen Cranley, McClaran, Jacqueline, Keyserlingk, Edward (1993) 'Adult children's perceptions of their responsibility to care for dependent elderly parents', *The Gerontologist*, vol 33, no 3, pp 315–23.

12: Drugs

Society invents a spurious convoluted logic tae absorb and change people whae's behaviour is outside its mainstream. Suppose that ah ken aw the pros and cons, know that ah'm gaunnae huv a short life, am ay sound mind etcetera, etcetera, but still want tae use smack? They won't let ye dae it. They won't let ye dae it, because it's seen as a sign ay thir ain failure. The fact that ye jist simply choose tae reject whit they huv tae offer. Choose us. Choose life. Choose mortgage payments; choose washing machines; choose cars; choose sitting oan a couch watching mind-numbing and spirit-crushing game shows, stuffing fucking junk food intae yir mooth. Choose rotting away, pishing and shiteing yersel in a home, a total fucking embarrassment tae the selfish, fucked-up brats ye've produced. Choose life.

Well, ah choose no tae choose life.

Irvine Welsh (1993) *Trainspotting*

In the words of one of the early Spanish visitors to the New World, 'they eat a root which they call peyote, and which they venerate as though it were a deity.'

233

Why they should have venerated it as a deity became apparent when such eminent psychologists as Jaensch, Havelock Ellis and Weir Mitchell began their experiments with mescalin, the active principle of peyote ... [A]ll concurred in assigning to mescalin a position among drugs of unique distinction. Administered in suitable doses, it changes the quality of consciousness more profoundly and yet is less toxic than any other substance in the pharmacologist's repertory ...

[O]ne one bright May morning, I swallowed four-tenths of a gram of mescalin dissolved in half a glass of water and sat down to wait for the results ...

Half an hour after swallowing the drug I became aware of a slow dance of golden lights. A little later there were sumptuous red surfaces swelling and expanding from bright nodes of energy that vibrated with a continuously changing, patterned life. At another time the closing of my eyes revealed a complex of gray structures, within which pale bluish spheres kept emerging into intense solidity and, having emerged, would slide noiselessly upwards, out of sight. But at no time were there faces or forms of men or animals. I saw no landscapes, no enormous spaces, no magical growth and metamorphosis of buildings, nothing remotely like a drama or a parable. The other world to which mescalin admitted me was not the world of visions; it existed out there, in what I could see with my eyes open. The great change was in the realm of objective fact. What had happened to my subjective universe was relatively unimportant.

I took my pill at eleven. An hour and a half later, I was sitting in my study, looking intently at a small glass vase. The vase contained only three flowers – a full-blown Belie of Portugal rose, shell pink with a hint at every petal's base of a hotter, flamier hue; a large magenta and cream-colored carnation; and, pale purple at the end of its broken stalk, the bold heraldic blossom of an iris. Fortuitous and provisional, the little nosegay broke all the rules of traditional good taste. At breakfast that morning I had been struck by the lively dissonance of its colors. But that was no longer the point. I was not looking now at an unusual flower arrangement. I was seeing what Adam had seen on the morning of his creation – the miracle, moment by moment, of naked existence ...

I continued to look at the flowers, and in their living light I seemed to detect the qualitative equivalent of breathing – but of a breathing without returns to a starting point, with no recurrent ebbs but only a repeated flow from beauty to heightened beauty, from deeper to ever deeper meaning. Words like 'grace' and 'transfiguration' came to my mind, and this, of course, was what, among other things, they stood for. My eyes travelled from the rose to the carnation, and from that feathery incandescence to the smooth scrolls of sentient amethyst which were the iris. The Beatific Vision, Sat Chit Ananda, Being-Awareness-Bliss – for the first time I understood, not on the verbal level, not by inchoate hints or at a distance, but precisely and completely what those prodigious syllables referred to.

Aldous Huxley (1954) *The Doors of Perception*

CASE STUDY 12.3

A few nights after meeting Roy and Herman, I used one of the syrettes, which was my first experience with junk. A syrette is like a toothpaste tube with a needle on the end. You push a pin down through the needle; the pin punctures the seal; and the syrette is ready to shoot.

Morphine hits the back of the legs first, then the back of the neck, a spreading wave of relaxation slackening the muscles away from the bones so that you seem to float without outlines like lying in warm salt water. As this relaxing wave spread through my tissues, I experienced a strong feeling of fear. I had the feeling that some horrible image was just beyond the field of vision, moving, as I turned my head, so that I never quite saw it. I felt nauseous; I lay down and closed my eyes. A series of pictures passed, like watching a movie: A huge neon-lighted cocktail bar that got larger and larger until streets, traffic, and street repairs were included in it; a waitress carrying a skull on a tray; stars in the clear sky. The physical impact of the fear of death; the shutting off of breath; the stopping of blood.

I dozed off and woke up with a start of fear. Next morning I vomited and felt sick until noon.

William Burroughs (1953) *Junkie*

The death of a 27-year-old mother of two who reacted badly to ecstasy highlights the risks of using the drug, a Sydney drug expert has warned. Meeghan Turra, from Mt Barker in the Adelaide Hills, died on Sunday after being rushed to hospital in the early hours of the morning. Relatives said it was the first time Ms Turra, who had two boys aged three and six months, had used ecstasy. They described her actions as completely out of character.

National Drug and Alcohol Research Council information officer Paul Dillon said Ms Turra was older than most people reported to have died from ecstasy.

'The interesting thing here is it was an older person', he said. 'Often when a young teen dies people say they had a lack of life experience and didn't know what they were doing, but she had some life experience. It would be very unusual if she died from MDMA poisoning but it could have been many different things, such as hypothermia or a pre-existing condition like a heart problem. It's interesting talking to groups of ecstasy users after someone dies. There's always a round of excuses why, but the reality is they died because they took ecstasy and it causes problems.'

Mr Dillon said recorded deaths from ecstasy use were rare, but they could be under-reported. 'It's very difficult to know the numbers because people often die a number of days after from complications so MDMA does not appear on the death certificate', he said.

David Braithwaite (2006) 'Mother's ecstasy death sparks warning', *Sydney Morning Herald*, 7 March

---

CASE STUDY 12.5

In 1919 US Congress passed the Volstead Act, prohibiting the manufacture, importation, sale and distribution of alcoholic beverages. The effects of the Act were so significant that a whole era in American history is named after it: Prohibition. The aim of Prohibition was to cut off the supply of alcohol and thereby reduce crime, ill-health, poverty and corruption. In the light of these aims Prohibition seems to have been in every respect a failure. While consumption of alcohol did diminish in the early years of Prohibition, by the time of its repeal in 1933 Americans were drinking as much as they had in 1919. The nature of that drinking, however, had changed. Obeying the so-called 'Iron Law of Prohibition', which states that the more intensely a law prohibiting a substance is enforced, the more potent the substance becomes, Americans now drank much greater quantities of hard liquor, and less wine and beer – and they paid more for what they drank. The potency of that liquor, produced in haste and secrecy, varied widely and unpredictably, as did its quality, with many instances of poisoning due to adulteration, hundreds of them fatal. Criminal gangs fought for control over the trade in alcohol and the riches that came with it (it is estimated that in his heyday as the crime lord of Chicago Al Capone was earning over $60 million a year from the sale of alcohol alone). Serious crime soared: murder rates nearly doubled through the Prohibition era, falling rapidly after repeal. Corruption was rampant: everyone from major politicians to the cop on the beat took bribes from bootleggers, crime bosses and owners of speakeasies [illegal bars]. Despite a vast increase in spending on law enforcement, the person in charge of enforcing the ban on alcohol, Commissioner of Prohibition Henry Anderson despairingly concluded that the effects of Prohibition included undermining of respect for the law in general, corrupting of public officials, and overburdening the court system.

Provided by the authors

CASE STUDY 12.6

I became a New York City policeman in 1956 and quickly became acquainted with problems of illegal drug use. I was assigned to Harlem. During the late 1950s, we cops watched in frustration as an epidemic of heroin addiction swept a community where limited opportunities created a fertile climate for escaping reality through drugs. Heroin took an awesome toll. Whole families and neighbourhoods seemed to fall to addiction. Street corners were filled with young men and women nodding on their feet like zombies. Under the influence of the powerful opiate, they abruptly jerked awake, alert for a few minutes before they again drifted off. Sometimes we responded to reports of an 'overdose' and found a muscular teenage boy DOA with the hypodermic needle still in his arm.

As a result of such experiences, cops were willing soldiers at the birth of the 'war on drugs'. (The term was first used by President Nixon in 1972.) The consequences of drug use were devastatingly clear to us. It seemed imperative that the government eradicate the 'plague' of addiction. We did what police do. We arrested everyone in sight when we saw a drug violation, and we saw them constantly. However, it did not take long to become disillusioned. Despite enormous increases in arrests, it was apparent that arrests did not cure users nor discourage pushers. The first thing addicts did when they got out of jail was to shoot up. And new pushers were dealing before the cell doors closed on their predecessors. It was easy for working cops to believe that lenient judges and an inefficient correctional system were at fault. After all, we were working hard, making drug arrests. But doubts were growing within the police ranks. We complained of inadequate laws and lenient sentences. The politicians responded.

Governor Nelson Rockefeller, who had presidential ambitions, convinced the New York State legislature to pass laws giving life sentences to drug sellers. To avoid life sentences, drug dealers recruited young boys who could only be charged with juvenile delinquency. The unintended consequence of the get tough policy was to create legions of teenage career criminals. Patrick V Murphy, the New York City police commissioner had opposed the legislation for this reason, but drug war fever prevailed among the politicians.

On the streets of Harlem we saw increases in violence stemming not from the use of heroin but from the commerce in heroin. Most of the users dozed away their lives and were incapable of violence. In Harlem, and other poor neighbourhoods, young boys who had dropped out of school and had little chance for legitimate careers suddenly saw more money than they had dreamed of and were willing to kill rivals who threatened their new affluence.

Notwithstanding our growing scepticism, we went about our

job. One day, my partner and I came across a drug user. That day, the addict we arrested was cooperative. He surrendered the needle hidden in his belt where it would be difficult to find. He pleaded with us. He was just a junkie. He couldn't take a bust right now. If we let him go he would 'give' us a pusher. He would make a drug buy and when he and the pusher went into a hallway to exchange money for drugs we would arrest the pusher in the act and let the addict go. To my surprise my partner agreed. Since he was senior, I reluctantly went along. We put the bottle cap and needle in the glove compartment of our police car and followed the addict. It was a warm summer day and there were lots of people on Lenox Ave as we coasted along, never more than ten feet from our prisoner. I had my hand on the door handle ready to bolt after him if he decided to break the agreement. But he was good to his word. He walked down the street talking to one person after another. The third dealer agreed to sell. When they went into a hallway we charged in and arrested the dealer. The addict 'escaped.'

It amazed me that in bright daylight the man had talked to pushers about buying illegal drugs with a marked police car and two uniformed policemen ten feet away. None of the men had been deterred by our presence. The first two dealers weren't being careful, they had already sold their supply. They found no reason to be hesitant. If we had not known what the addict was doing, we would have guessed they were talking about cars, girlfriends, sports, politics, or other innocent things.

For the first time, I realized how truly ineffective the police are in preventing drug use through enforcement of criminal statutes. Unlike traditional mala-in-se crimes (wrong in themselves) where a victim who is robbed or assaulted comes to the police and criminal justice system for redress and protection, drug dealing and drug use are confidential, consensual transactions between people who treasure their privacy. Everyday, hundreds of thousands, perhaps millions of drug crimes occur and the police have no way of knowing about them, let alone the ability to prevent them. Consequently, the potential of being arrested and punished is far less than in other crimes and is not a credible deterrent. And, of course, truly hard-core drug users discount the threat of arrest in proportion to their need for drugs.

Adapted from Joseph D McNamara (1999) 'The war the police didn't declare and can't win', 5 October

CASE STUDY 12.7

'A drugs-free world – we can do it!' That is the official slogan of the UN's current 10-year war-on-drugs strategy. A drugs summit marking the halfway point in that 10-year plan ended in Vienna last week – and it has all been a triumphant success. Or so said the director of the UN office on drugs and crime in his breezy opening address. 'Does drug control policy work?' he asked rhetorically. 'This question can be answered in the affirmative and unanimously.' Yes, the UN programme is 'on target to reach its goals' – to eradicate drug abuse and the cultivation of coca, cannabis and opium by the year 2008. Yes, really.

It was a breathtaking lie which everyone in the hall knew was nonsense – and he knew they knew it. Out there, drug prices are still falling and drug use is generally thought to be increasing. A few optimistic experts say it has stabilised – but few believe it. In Britain, the national treatment agency says addiction is rising by 7% a year. Drugs continue to cause political disintegration in poor producer countries at the hands of international crime, while causing social mayhem among the poor in rich consumer countries.

The only permissible line decreed in three UN conventions is a 'Just Say No' policy. All countries signing the conventions must enforce total prohibition laws, so no delegate could question whether it works. Afghanistan's crop this year will be back up to pre-Taliban levels – providing 90% of heroin: the country has no other export and the growers are far beyond the reach of Kabul's feeble authority. Colombia's US-imposed crackdown on coca has lead to huge planting in Bolivia and Peru instead ...

In Britain the government has moved with caution, not through any liberal instinct but under the sheer pressure of failure. The official guesstimate of the cost of drug addiction is somewhere between £10bn and £18bn a year – mostly in crime and its consequences: each addict is estimated to steal £13 000 a year to survive. Policy now centres on the 250 000 hard drug users reckoned to cause most of the crime. The government has greatly expanded treatment programmes: by 2008 most will have treatment. Yet still only half the addicts in prison get treatment – which is a mad false economy. Drug treatment pays for itself three to four times over.

Comparisons between countries are tricky. The Netherlands has had phenomenal success, with heroin addiction falling. Addicts are a shrinking and ageing group, well supervised and under control. Is that due to a good, well-financed, rational treatment programme? More likely it is due to the structure of Dutch life, a far more equal society with an absence of gross poverty. Those western societies such as Britain and the US, with the greatest wealth gap and the most poverty, have the worst drug problems: it is an affliction of poverty among affluence … Ending poverty would be the best cure, among both the western consumers and the third world growers.

But second best would be an end to a global policy that turns drugs from a manageable disease of the few into a widescale social calamity. Prohibition has followed the same predictable course as the US experiment in banning alcohol: it breeds crime. If methadone or heroin were prescribed by doctors globally to all addicts, drug-fuelled crime would fall.

Polly Toynbee (2003) 'Just say no to a drugs policy that doesn't work', *The Guardian*, 23 April

ETHICAL ANALYSIS

What is a drug?

In this chapter when we use the word 'drugs' we are referring to psychoactive substances. That means that when ingested they affect mental functioning through, for example, elevating or depressing mood, or changing normal modes of thinking or perceiving the external world or one's own body.

Many drugs have medical uses, as pain killers for example: moral controversies concerning drug use focus on the non-medicinal use of drugs. In every society people use drugs for many purposes, ranging from social lubrication, to spiritual enlightenment, to recreational intoxication. In modern societies illicit drugs such as marijuana, cocaine, ecstasy and so on are widely used. That these drugs are so extensively – and in many cases, unashamedly used (see case study 12.1) – itself raises a range of issues, such as the justification for legally prohibiting behaviour which is both common and widely accepted and which, moreover, seems to affect only the person who is engaging in it. We discuss this question below, but the problems concerning the non-medical use of drugs are not confined to illegal drugs. In modern Western societies, for example, the three most commonly used drugs (in order of usage) are caffeine, alcohol and nicotine, all of which are legal.

The very term 'drug' has taken on a pejorative overtone: we hear of the 'War on Drugs', the menace of drugs, and so on. It is worth, then, making the obvious, but apparently easily overlooked, point that drugs are in a variety of ways good. At the very least, they satisfy the desires of many people. Of course, since those desires may be trivial, or depraved, or irrational, that fact alone may not seem to provide very weighty support for the value of drugs. However, much drug use is valuable, not just because users want to engage in it, but because it provides real benefits. We can feel more alert after drinking a cup of coffee, more relaxed after a glass of wine, and perhaps more enlightened as a result of taking mescalin (see case study 12.2). Furthermore, drug taking is in the first instance a self-regarding action. No doubt, someone's drug taking will often lead to behaviour which will adversely affect others, as when they drink large amounts of alcohol then drive recklessly. But while driving after drinking is obviously a morally bad thing, it does not follow that drinking in itself is. Of course, the fact that something is a self-regarding action does not put it beyond moral assessment or criticism, but generally we hold that individuals should be allowed to act as they wish in matters that only directly affect them, and furthermore that the individual is typically in the best position to judge what is in their own best interests.

Given that drug taking is a self-regarding activity, if it is also accepted that it is, or can be, beneficial to the consumer, then it would seem that the burden of justification falls on those who see drug taking as morally bad. Before considering the kinds of arguments that are put forward to attempt to support that claim, it is worth noting that few people believe that all kinds of non-medicinal use of drugs are morally problematic. Even if substances such as caffeine are, strictly speaking drugs, there do seem to be important differences between them and 'harder' drugs, such as heroin or alcohol. Moreover, there is also an important difference between, say, occasionally drinking a few glasses of beer with work-mates on Friday afternoon, and drinking oneself to a state of unconsciousness every night.

The core of moral concerns about drugs is their addictive nature. Many drugs are habit forming: the person who uses them over a period of time tends to want to go on using them. But addiction is more than habit. Many drugs, used over a period of time, create dependency: the user cannot function without them. The brain has a natural capacity to produce mood elevating chemicals given the right stimuli. Drugs such as heroin provide an artificial stimulus for their production. Taking such drugs regularly lessens the capacity of the brain to produce mood elevating chemicals of its own accord. Hence a dose of a drug that would have produced a feeling of euphoria in a novice user, serves only to bring the experienced user to a point of normality. In other words the regular user develops a tolerance for the drug; they need greater and greater amounts (perhaps up to some plateau) to produce the same effect. The changes in brain chemistry consequent on regular drug use also means that stopping regular use will produce mental and physical pain until the brain returns to full functioning, that is the regular user will experience withdrawal symptoms.

Drugs can be ranked in terms of addictiveness according to the intensity of their effects, degree of tolerance and severity of withdrawal. A drug such as caffeine is relatively low in the intensity of its effect, and tolerance levels, while withdrawal symptoms are minor. Hence it is a weakly addictive drug. Heroin, on the other hand, is a high intensity, high tolerance level drug, with extreme withdrawal symptoms, so it is a strongly addictive drug.

The medical model

Addiction is morally problematic for a range of reasons. One of the most important concerns about addiction focusses on the way it impairs autonomy. However, how drug addiction affects autonomy is not as straightforward as many popular and academic discussions make out. Often drug addiction is presented in popular films and novels as a condition in which the need for the drug has become a kind of basic and overriding drive. The drug user has lost all capacity to choose whether to seek out and use the drug; they have become a kind of puppet, controlled by their addiction.

Such a view of addiction is also at the basis of the so-called 'medical model' of addiction. This sees drug addiction as, or akin to, a disease or other medical condition. Treatment for addicts ought to take the form appropriate to a medical condition. Like being infected with a fever, drug addiction, on this view, is not a moral condition, and the drug addict's use of drugs is not something for which the drug addict is morally responsible. (Although, if the medical analogy is to be preserved, the drug addict can be held morally responsible for failing to take drug treatment (assuming it is available).) Accordingly, so the argument runs, the drug addict is not a fit object of praise or blame, and the appropriate treatment is some form of medical or quasi-medical – especially therapeutic – intervention, such as placing a heroin addict in a methadone program. What is ruled out in this picture is blaming the addict and making negative moral judgments about the addict's addiction. It makes no more sense to condemn an addict for their continued use of their favoured drug than it does to blame a polio victim for their inability to run.

This view of addiction, then, has it that the addict's autonomy has been destroyed, at least in respect of their drug-related behaviour. But this view is dubious (Levy 2006). To say that someone is autonomous (in some area of their life) implies that they are capable of recognising, assessing, and responding to reasons. If, as the medical model implies, drug addicts have had their autonomy in respect of their drug use destroyed, it follows that they are completely incapable of doing this. Note that the fact that addicts tend to persist in their drug taking (and the activities which are necessary to do so) does not in itself show that they are not acting autonomously, since as we noted above, the relief offered by taking drugs and the pains of withdrawal consequent on stopping are powerful reasons for them to persist. That is, the costs of stopping may be calculated to be greater than the benefits of so doing. This does not prove that addicts continue to take drugs because they make an autonomous choice to do so, but it does indicate that their actions are at least compatible with autonomous choice.

To determine whether addicts are acting autonomously we would need to possess compelling factual evidence indicating that addicts are (or are not) capable of recognising and responding to reasons. We now possess a good deal of evidence that indicates drug addicts can and do remain responsive to reasons regarding their drug use, and as the balance of such reasons changes, so can their behaviour. For example, it is not uncommon for young women who are addicted to heroin to stop using it upon falling pregnant. Clearly these women realise that if they continue to take heroin through their pregnancy they will damage their unborn babies. The (moral) desire not to do so is a sufficient motivator for them to stop using heroin despite the costs of doing so.

If this explanation is accepted then it follows that drug addicts do not totally lose their autonomy in relation to their drug use simply in virtue of their addiction, and the medical model at least in its pure form, should be rejected. Rather, we can and should continue to see the drug user as a member of the moral community, a person whom it is appropriate to direct moral appeals to and to make moral judgments about. Indeed, much of our actual practice and responses to drug addicts only makes sense if we see addicts in this way. Even proponents of the medical model implicitly appeal to such moral considerations in their practice, which often aims to help addicts change their attitudes through counselling and the like. Such methods depend on the addict understanding and accepting that his addiction is undesirable; that is, *morally* undesirable. Furthermore, we are (and should be) prepared to praise someone who manages to overcome their addiction, such as the pregnant women discussed above.

Even if we accept that drug addicts are not beyond the realm of moral considerations, there may still be good reasons to be careful about the expression of moral judgments on them (Miller 2006). Perhaps, for example, it is therapeutically desirable for drug counsellors to suspend moral judgments about their addict clients in order to maximise the chances of successful treatment. Or more broadly for members of the community to resist stigmatising drug addicts for fear that this will reinforce the factors that support their addiction. But moral judgments may still be appropriate here, even if their open expression might not be.

Drugs, morality and law

We have argued against the claim that drug addicts totally lose their autonomy in relation to their drug use, simply in virtue of their addiction. Nevertheless, one of the main reasons for thinking that drug addiction is morally undesirable is because of its adverse effect on autonomy. As a preliminary to our argument here, we need to point out that the adjective 'autonomous' can be applied to people, or to the choices that people make, or the lives that they lead. When we talk about a person being autonomous, we mean that they are self-determining, in the sense that they can decide what is important and valuable to them, and possess the capacity to make reason-based choices on the basis of knowledge of relevant facts (as discussed in Chapter 7). When we talk about someone leading an autonomous life, we mean both that it is a life lived by an autonomous person, and that it offers scope for reason-based choice and some realistic chance of obtaining the things the person takes to be valuable. To see the difference between these senses of 'autonomous' think of someone who is sentenced to a period of solitary confinement in an authoritarian prison. The prisoner may still be described as autonomous – even though there is almost no scope for the exercise of choice in his daily existence – that is, his life at this point lacks autonomy.

In terms of this distinction our argument is that a drug addict does not lose her status as an autonomous person just in virtue of her addiction. Nevertheless, she is likely to lead a life of diminished autonomy. To the extent to which her life must be structured to accommodate her addiction, the range of choices which is open to her to explore and express her values becomes progressively narrower. Moreover, possessing the capacity for autonomy and living an autonomous life are intertwined. Just as one can only live an autonomous life if one is an autonomous person, so one can only become and remain an autonomous person if there is sufficient scope to live an autonomous life. A long-standing addiction, then, is likely to diminish the addict's autonomy.

Autonomy is good in itself, so a loss of autonomy is bad in itself. But autonomy is also valuable in that it is a necessary condition for gaining other goods. The loss of autonomy is bad in that it removes the possibility of attaining these goods. The long-term addict whose life is centred on her addiction to the extent that she loses any interest in maintaining deep human relationships such as friendships, or in pursuing projects which express and extend her talents, simply ends up living in a largely solipsistic world. This consists of her experiencing by herself an ongoing cycle of drug-induced cravings and 'highs'. For rational, social animals, such as human beings, this is surely an impoverished existence, and therefore ethically undesirable.

Abuse of drugs, then, is a serious problem for the abuser in virtue of its effect on her autonomy. It also tends to produce other ill-effects such as mental and physical ill-health and even death. Drug abuse also generates a range of social problems, including violence and family breakdown (especially in the case of alcohol). Given the scale and severity of drug abuse in societies such as Australia, attempting to limit the abuse of these substances, then, is a legitimate aim of public policy.

One of the tools used for reducing substance abuse is the legal prohibition of the sale, possession or use of certain recreational drugs, such as heroin, cocaine and marijuana. The criminalisation of recreational drug use poses, at least on the face of it, a problem for any theory which sees personal autonomy as of central importance. Firstly, when a person uses a recreational drug they do not, simply in virtue of that use, violate the rights of anyone else (hence drug use is often referred to as a 'victimless crime'). Secondly, preventing someone from using a drug of their choice, or penalising them when they do so, actually seems to violate their right to autonomy. (For a thorough discussion of the pros and cons of making drug use illegal, see Husak and de Marneffe (2005).)

Nevertheless, making and enforcing laws against recreational drugs can be justified. As noted above, the abuse of such drugs has a range of bad effects, which are themselves likely to involve, or lead to, serious abuse of the rights of others. Further, as we have argued, addictive drugs such as heroin can seriously undermine addicts' autonomy. Hence the prohibition of recreational drugs can be justified both in terms of the aim of reducing the bad effects that are consequent on their use, and in terms of the protection and promotion of autonomy. Understanding the point of the legal prohibition of drugs as being to prevent and minimise the harms of abusing such drugs has important implications for the way such laws (and more broadly the range of social policies aiming to control drug use) are framed and enforced. In particular, legislation should be informed by that aim, and we should be alert to how poorly conceived laws or clumsily executed policing can exacerbate, rather than reduce, harm (Bronitt and McSherry 2001). The American experiment of 'Prohibition' in the 1920s is instructive in this respect. (See case study 12.5.) The legal prohibition of the sale of alcohol in the USA in the 1920s aimed to reduce the evils that flowed from misuse of alcohol. As well as failing in this aim – perversely, Prohibition seems to have contributed to a growth in problem drinking, and the clandestine production of poorly made alcohol led to a huge increase in poisonings – Prohibition fuelled a massive upsurge in serious crime as criminals fought over the lucrative trade in illicit liquor, and in corruption of public officials (see case studies 12.6

and 12.7 for descriptions of similar perverse outcomes in the modern 'war against drugs').

On the so-called 'harm minimisation' approach to recreational drugs, an important distinction needs to be drawn between those who use such drugs, and those who supply them. Drug users are not themselves, as discussed above, engaging in action that is itself harmful to others. Policies directed at users, then, should be primarily aimed to divert them from engaging in drug use. Over-aggressive attempts to, say, arrest and prosecute drug users can have unintended harmful side effects – for example by leading to greater use of shared needles by intravenous drug users who are unwilling to carry drug injecting equipment for fear of drawing police attention – and do little or nothing to reduce the use of drugs by such people. On the other hand, drug sellers *are* themselves engaging in activity which harms others, so there is no in principle objection to using the full force of the law to stop them from doing this, and to punish them for having done so. Furthermore, drug sellers are often engaged in other criminal activities. Nevertheless, policies directed to both sellers and users of illicit drugs should be sensitive to empirical evidence concerning their effectiveness in reducing both demand and supply of illicit substances. It is at least conceivable that legalisation and supervision of presently illicit substances would be better in consequentialist terms than continued criminalisation.

Readings

Braithwaite, David (2006) 'Mother's ecstasy death sparks warning', *Sydney Morning Herald*, 7 March, available at <http://www.smh.com.au> (accessed 21/2/09).

Bronitt, Simon and McSherry, Bernadette (2001) *Principles of Criminal Law*, Law Book Co, Sydney, Ch 15.

Burroughs, William (1953) *Junkie*, New English Library, London, pp 14–15.

Husak, Douglas and de Marneffe, Peter (2005) *The Legalization of Drugs*, Cambridge University Press, Cambridge.

Huxley, Aldous (1954) *The Doors of Perception*, Chatto & Windus Ltd, London, available at <http://www.psychedelic-library.org/doors.htm> (accessed 23/1/09).

Levy, Neil (2006) 'Autonomy and addiction', *Canadian Journal of Philosophy*, vol 36, no 3, pp 427–48.

McNamara, Joseph D (1999) 'The war the police didn't declare and can't win', Cato Institute, 5 October, available at <http://www.cato.org/realaudio/

drugwar/papers/mcnamara.html> (accessed 23/1/09).

Miller, Seumas (2006) 'Privacy, confidentiality and the treatment of drug addicts' in Kleinig, John and Einstein, Stanley (eds) *Ethical Challenges for Intervening in Drug Use*, Office of International Criminal Justice, Huntsville, Texas, pp 465–81.

National Commission on Law Observance and Enforcement (1931) *Enforcement of the Prohibition Laws of the United States*, Government Printing Office, Washington.

Toynbee, Polly (2003) 'Just say no to a drugs policy that doesn't work', *The Guardian*, 23 April, available at <http://www.guardian.co.uk> (accessed 21/2/09).

Welsh, Irvine (1993) *Trainspotting*, Secker & Warburg, London, pp 187–88.

Yaffe, Gideon (2002) 'Recent work on addiction and responsible agency', *Philosophy and Public Affairs*, vol 30, no 2.

13: Corruption

For years a bitter dispute raged between the two men who both claimed to have been the discoverer of the virus that causes AIDS, the American Robert Gallo, Head of the National Institute of Health's Laboratory of Tumor Cell Biology, and the Frenchman, Luc Montagnier of the Pasteur Institute. More than personal pride was involved, it became a matter of institutional and even national prestige. In the late 1980s Gallo finally conceded that the virus he identified (in work done in 1983 and 1984) was from a sample contaminated by a sample sent to him by Montagnier. A National Institute of Health Investigation found Gallo's report of the work full of falsifications of date and misrepresentations of method.

It is in this context that we should examine the actions of Dr Michael Garretta, former Head of the National Blood Transfusion Centre in France. In the spring of 1985 it was clear that the French supplies of a blood-clotting substance needed by haemophiliacs was contaminated by the AIDS virus. French haemophiliacs could have been protected if then-available techniques for decontaminating blood tainted with HIV had been used, or if the tainted supplies had been replaced. The technology was developed in the United States.

251

So, either way, the French would have been relying on American science – something that the French government was loath to do, especially given the dispute between the two countries over the discovery of the AIDS virus – and the cost would have been substantial (one estimate put it at $40 million).

Although Garetta was aware of these possibilities, he ordered that the supplies be used until they were exhausted. (They were withdrawn in October 1985, after the French decontamination process was available.) As a result, some 1500 haemophiliacs were infected; at least 300 have since died. In October 1992, Dr Garetta was convicted of 'fraudulent description of goods' in the distribution of tainted blood, and sentenced to four years in prison (the maximum allowed). In Garetta's defence, it was argued that his superiors were aware of the dangers and that he acted as an agent within a bureaucracy committed to safeguarding the prestige of French science. In short, he was fulfilling his role responsibilities.

Adapted from Daniel E Wueste (ed) (1994) *Ethics and Social Responsibility*

CASE STUDY 13.2

A prison officer, the popular and well-thought-of 'Officer Bob', is within weeks of retirement, at the end of a long and well-considered career as a custodial officer in the state's prison service. Another custodial officer, new to the service, has remarked that on occasion Bob appears to vague-out, and his manner with inmates is sometimes too familiar for this observer's tastes. Bob's workmates defend him, citing the recent death of Bob's wife, his imminent retirement, and other considerations attracting compassion. The new officer is informed, 'He is still the best officer on the shift' and, fearful of attracting workmate resentment, he says nothing further against Bob.

Later, the new officer is on duty in Prison Block G at 10:00 pm, the time when prisoners are returned to their cells and locked-in for the night. He is checking the utility closet in G block, ensuring the block's cleaning supplies have been put away, when he glances through the window.

There is a clear view through the window of the utility closet to H Block, which is opposite, its layout a mirror-image of G block, and he observes Officer Bob standing in the G Block utility cupboard in close proximity to a prisoner. Brown, the G Block prisoner, bears the reputation of being a homosexual, and an inmate who engages in drug-dealing within the prison. Bob is observed to reach into his pocket and withdraw a small brown-paper package which he gives to the inmate. Both men are smiling and Brown accepts the package and in return embraces Bob and kisses him full on the mouth before departing.

As he stands in indecision at the window of the utility cupboard, the new Officer is astonished to see Officer Bob and the prisoner Brown re-enter the 'H' Block utility cupboard at a time well-past lock-down. They produce drug apparatus and both appear to engage in inhaling a white substance from a phial. They then extinguish the lights in the cupboard and sink to the floor, below the level of sight from G Block. Shocked, the new officer backs out of the G Block utility cupboard, to unexpectedly confront his supervisor, Lieutenant Davis who, remarking [on] his shocked expression, inquires if anything is amiss.

The new officer, aware that Bob is seriously, perhaps even criminally, compromised by his actions, nevertheless hesitates. Had his eyes deceived him? If he repeated what he saw to a person in authority, would he be believed? What action should he next take?

Bernard J McCarthy (1991) 'Keeping an eye on the keeper: prison corruption and its control'

CASE STUDY 13.3

In what has come to be known in Australia as the 'Cash for Comment' case, John Laws, a well-known Australian radio celebrity with an audience of two million listeners, made an agreement with a number of banks that he would provide favourable comment on the banking sector, if the banks paid him the sum of A$1.2 million. This financial transaction between Laws and the banks was carried out in secret; in particular, it was concealed from the public, including his audience. Just a few weeks prior to making this deal, Laws had used his air-time to repeatedly criticise the banks; he claimed that they were acting unethically by imposing unjustified fees on their customers, and cutting back on vital services.

Provided by the authors

CASE STUDY 13.4

HIH was the second largest insurance company in Australia, and it collapsed in March 2001 with debts of A$5.3 billion. At the time of its collapse, some two million HIH policy holders were adversely affected. Up until the mid-1990s, HIH had focussed upon liability insurance, at one stage holding 50 percent of major insurance risks in Australia. As a result of a number of business factors (the advent of class actions, lawyers' contingency fees, and a 25 percent increase per annum growth in claims), HIH sought to broaden its insurance base by a series of purchases of other insurance enterprises. As a result of a disastrous buying spree, HIH's equity holdings fell from a healthy 17 percent in 1993 to six percent in 1998. Long before HIH went into liquidation, its losses were widely known.

Prior to HIH's collapse, the Australian government, conscious of the impact upon the economy of the failure of the company, agreed to what turned out to be a futile rescue package of A$640 million. The collapse of HIH had such an adverse impact upon the Australian insurance industry that the government undertook a Royal Commission into the reasons for the collapse, including why the regime of corporate and insurance regulation failed so spectacularly.

The Australian corporate regulators laid charges against the CEO, Ray Williams, a former non-executive director, Rodney Adler, and the chief finance officer, Dominic Fodera. While the root causes of HIH's collapse were bad business decisions, a number of parties were alleged to have been involved in corrupt practices. The CEO was charged with having recklessly and dishonestly borrowed large amounts, in the knowledge that the company was insolvent. He was also charged with neglecting his director's duties by making business-decisions which failed the test of good faith and proper use of company resources. In one deal, HIH purchased Pacific Eagle Equities for A$10 million. That entity was a family-owned company of Rodney Adler who then allegedly committed an offence under the *Corporations Act* by manipulating the stock market in buying A$4 million of HIH shares in Pacific Eagle Equities' name.

The complex dealing between Ray Williams and Rodney Adler included the purchase of FAI Insurance, a company in which Adler had significant interests. FAI held interests in a company called Home Security International. Adler allegedly arranged to have a US investor buy 48000 shares in Home Security International which caused a 30 percent 'spike' in the value of the stock. As a result of this deal, A$12 million was added to FAI's value and, soon after, the company posted a yearly profit of A$8.6 million. As a result of this profit, the price paid by HIH for FAI when it purchased the company was far in excess of its true value.

The Royal Commission into HIH found that, as the company lurched towards collapse, it engaged in corporate excesses involving travel, entertainment, charitable donations, and executive gifts. These excesses stripped over A$32 million out of its assets. Staff were given gold watches, and a tip of A$700 was paid at a dinner attended by the CEO and HIH executives at Port Douglas (Port Douglas is an expensive tropical resort some 1500 miles away from Sydney, where HIH was based). Just weeks before the collapse, A$180000 was paid to a Melbourne football club which was in some financial difficultly.

The HIH collapse has sparked a lively debate into the ethical responsibility of company directors and the role of corporate regulators. The laying of charges against the principal parties has been widely applauded by the media. The corporate regulators, particularly the Australian Prudential Regulation Authority, claims that it was profoundly misled by HIH, and thus it, in turn, had inadvertently misled the government about the seriousness of the crisis facing the company. The federal Opposition has questioned how the collapse was not anticipated by the regulatory authorities, given the amount of material showing that HIH was in trouble up to two years before the collapse.

Seumas Miller, Peter Roberts and Edward Spence (2005)
Corruption and Anti-corruption

CASE STUDY 13.5

[Detective Robert Leuci was a member of New York Police Department (NYPD) Narcotics Division's Special Investigative Unit (SIU). SIU Detectives, although junior grade, were acknowledged as the force's most expert drug investigators. In an addicted city, increasingly victimised by drug-related crime, their head-line grabbing, multi-million drug busts, turning in suitcases, a steamer trunk, once a whole closet full of drugs, earned universal approbation; the city fathers tagged them 'Princes of the City'.

There was an elitism and a positive esprit de corps in the SIU; together with a solidaristic tendency that defeated supervision, the NYPD didn't look too closely at the unit's modus operandi, ends-justified by a stream of high-profile arrests that reflected credit on the remainder of a department otherwise not enjoying good press. Working with a patently corrupt legal system, amongst suspects lost to the moral pressures of normal society, the SIU's autonomous four-man teams pursued their investigations in an ecology of moral ambiguity: a place where values collide. Beyond the ethical command of even their own tainted force, their methods descended into the same order of criminality they sought to suppress.

Leuci was undergoing a personal crisis; a younger brother's previously undetected narcotics habit; his father's recognition of his and his workmates' corruption. He began to unburden himself to Nicholas Scopetta, a prosecutor from the Commission to Investigate Alleged Police Corruption – the 'Knapp Commission'. Part of the text of an initial contact, including Leuci's apologia pro vita sua, is reproduced here.]

'You people of the Knapp Commission', he said, 'are focusing on the Police Department. You tell cops that you are out to catch them taking meals, taking Christmas presents, giving drugs to junkies. It's absolutely incredible. Cops are looking at you and saying: You absolute bastards. It's you guys, the assistant district attorneys, lawyers, judges who run the system, and the whole fucking thing from top to bottom is corrupt. We know how you become a judge. You pay $50 000 and you become a judge. We see stores open on Sunday on Fifth Avenue, but they can't be open in Little Italy. The only people that know us, care for us, love us, are other cops. You people are just looking to hurt us. You want to lay on us the responsibility for fucking up the system.'

'Do you know what it's like to be a narcotics detective?' Leuci continued, 'Do you have any conception? Do you know what it's like on a February night in South Brooklyn a block from the piers with two addict informants in the back of the car, both of them crying, begging you for a bag of heroin? Do you know what it's like going home fifty miles away, and getting a phone call five minutes after you're home saying, I blew the shot, please come back and give me another bag. And driving fifty miles back in and watching him tie up and walking out of the room. Then working with him the next morning and locking up some dope pusher that's just as sick as he is. It's an insanity. And going into the office and the lieutenant says you have to make five arrests this month. Do you know what it's like working six, seven days a week? You have to be one of the best, otherwise you go back to swinging a stick.' ...

'You're in Westbury, or West End Avenue', Leuci ranted on. 'We're in El Barrio, we're on 15th Street. You want us to keep everybody inside the barricades so you can stay outside. I'm on Pleasant Avenue and 116th Street at three o'clock in the morning, just me and my partner and Tony somebody that we have been following for three weeks, and he's going to offer me money, and me and my partner are going to decide whether we'll take it or not. You don't care about me and some black revolutionary is going to whack me out if he gets a chance, some newspaper is going to call me a thief whether

I do it or I don't do it. The only one who cares about me is my partner. It's me and him and this guy we caught. We're going to take him
to jail and lock him up. We're going to take his money. Fuck him, fuck
you, fuck them … I see what kind of man you are and I see what kind
of man my partner is and there's no comparison, see? I'm going to
side with him. He tells me it's okay Bobby, hey Bobby, it's you and
me against the world. You guys are eating in the Copa six nights a
week. We try to get sixty dollars expense money, and the department won't even give us that.'

Leuci swallowed painfully. 'You're winning in the end anyway.
We're selling ourselves, our families. These people we take money
from own us. Our family's future rests on the fact that some dope-
pusher is not going to give us up, or some killer, some total piece of
shit, is not going to give us up.'

Robert Daley (2005) Prince of the City

CASE STUDY 13.6

A social worker, Bill Fenton, has been working in a residential
facility for adults with severe physical disabilities for a number of
years. He loves the job and has succeeded in organising a Residents'
Committee, securing employment or tertiary education for many
of the residents, and reuniting several residents with their families
so that regular visits are now held. Generally, Bill has seen his job
as 'opening up' the residential from being a closed institution run
as a 'hospital' to being an accommodation facility which is more
home-like.

Eighteen months ago, Bill was part of an interview panel which
appointed a new Director of Nursing, Gary Keith. In the last year,
Gary has actively assisted Bill in his task of 'normalising' the nursing
home. Staff no longer wear uniforms, residents participate in making
the rules, Gary has even approved alterations to the facility so that
residents can have their own bedrooms and privacy. Since these
alterations were completed, two of the residents have announced
their engagement.

Bill has been delighted with the co-operation he has received from Gary. Although Gary is technically his 'supervisor' and he is accountable to Gary as Director of Nursing for his work at the residential facility, Bill finds that Gary supports the work he does. Gary leaves Bill to work as an independent professional, something which has not always happened with previous directors of nursing with whom he was often in conflict over how the residential should be run. During the last 18 months, Bill and Gary have also become friends, playing squash on a weekly basis and often socialising with each other and their families at weekends.

One Friday afternoon, Bill is approached by a delegation from the residents' committee. They tell Bill that they believe that several of the residents are being double charged for bills that they are sure they have already paid or part paid. They report that this began about 12 months ago, first with only one or two residents who assumed it was their own mistake. Recently however, several residents have discovered that 'quite a few' people thought that they had been double charged for rent. In addition, bank balances seem to have changed, with residents noting small but frequent withdrawals from their accounts which they do not remember requesting.

Most of the residents have lived at the residential facility for many years and this sort of thing had never happened before. Traditionally the Director of Nursing has access to the residents' accounts as the local bank is not physically accessible. Rent cheques made out by the residents to the organisation are banked by Gary, who also makes withdrawals at the request of the residents. The Residents' Committee is concerned that they are being 'ripped off' by the new Director of Nursing. The delegation from the Residents' Committee asks Bill for help with what to do next. Bill is about to go out for drinks with Gary who has told him that he wants to discuss the possibility of promoting Bill.

Provided by Wendy Bowles

A young officer, Joe, seeks advice from the police chaplain. Joe is working with an experienced detective, Mick, who is also Joe's brother-in-law, and looked up to by Joe as a good detective who gets results. Joe and Mick are working on a case involving a known drug-dealer and paedophile. Joe describes his problem as follows:

> Father – he has got a mile of form, including getting kids hooked on drugs, physical and sexual assault on minors, and more. Anyway, surveillance informed Mick that the drug-dealer had just made a buy. As me and Mick approached the drug-dealer's penthouse flat we noticed a parcel come flying out the window of the flat onto the street. It was full of heroin. The drug-dealer was in the house, but we found no drugs inside. Mick thought it would be more of a sure thing if we found the evidence in the flat rather than on the street – especially given the number of windows in the building. The defence would find it more difficult to deny possession. Last night Mick tells me that he was interviewed and signed a statement that we both found the parcel of heroin under the sink in the flat. He said all I had to do was to go along with the story in court and everything will be sweet, no worries. What should I do Father – perjury is a serious criminal offence.

Provided in a suitably disguised form by Father Jim Boland, chaplain to the New South Wales Police

ETHICAL ANALYSIS

Corruption in any institution or profession is highly problematic, since it tends to undermine the institution or profession, and corrodes the moral character of institutional actors and professional practitioners. Such undermining and corrosion inevitably, over time, reduce the likelihood that the institutions and professions in question will achieve their basic purposes.

Varieties of corruption

Corruption is exemplified by a diverse array of phenomena (Miller 2005, Miller et al 2005):

- A national leader accepts bribes.
- A political party secures a majority vote by arranging for ballot boxes to be stuffed with false voting papers.
- A businessman borrows heavily notwithstanding the fact that he knows his company is insolvent (case study 13.4).
- A journalist provides unwarranted favourable comment about the banking sector in return for financial rewards from that sector (case study 13.3).
- Another journalist consistently provides unwarranted unfavourable comment about a political party in order to influence the electorate against that party.
- A police officer fabricates evidence to secure convictions (case study 13.7).
- A medical research administrator engages in fraudulent descriptions of blood supplies. He knows that they are contaminated, and then orders that they be used, notwithstanding the dangers in so doing. All this in order to protect the reputation of his research work (case study 13.1).
- A number of doctors close ranks and refuse to testify against a colleague who they know has been negligent in relation to an unsuccessful surgical operation leading to loss of life.
- A prisoner provides sexual favours to a corrections officer in exchange for drugs (case study 13.2).
- An actor provides sexual favours to film directors in exchange for acting roles.
- A respected researcher's success relies on plagiarising the work of others.
- A public official in charge of allocating community

housing to needy citizens unfairly discriminates against a minority group he despises.

- A manager only promotes those who ingratiate themselves to her.
- A sports trainer provides banned substances to the athletes he trains, in order to enhance their performance.

There are many *institutional* forms of corruption, for example, in the political, law enforcement, judicial, business, medical and academic areas, to name only some. There are at least as many institutional forms of corruption as there are human institutions that might become corrupted.

Many *offence types* are considered acts of corruption, for example, bribery, fabricating evidence (police), plagiarism (academic), lying under oath (doctor to protect colleagues) or in order to ruin reputations (journalist), abusing one's authority to gain sexual favours (social worker in relation to client). What do these have in common? What is the definition of corruption?

Many cases of corruption also involve unlawful activities. But some do not:

- It might not be unlawful for an actor to provide sexual favours to film directors in exchange for roles in movies.
- In 2001 it was not unlawful for Sydney-based talkback radio host and commentator, John Laws, to receive cash for comment; Laws and some Australian bankers struck a deal whereby he was to be paid to refrain from pejorative criticism of the banking sector. (See case study 13.3.)
- Prior to 1977 it was not unlawful for US companies to offer bribes to secure foreign contracts.

Therefore corrupt actions are not necessarily unlawful actions. Why not? Because corruption is not fundamentally a matter of law, rather it is a matter of morality.

Some laws are morally bad, for example, the racially discriminatory laws in apartheid South Africa or in Nazi Germany were morally bad. Perhaps the law banning euthanasia under all circumstances is bad. (See Chapter 9.) Some morally good practices are not enshrined in laws. It is morally good for parents to be kind to their children, but there is no law to this effect.

Corrupt actions are immoral actions. But not all immoral actions are corrupt actions; corruption is only one species of immorality. Consider an otherwise gentle husband who in a fit of anger strikes his adulterous wife and kills her. The husband has committed a morally wrong act, but not an act of corruption.

Similarly, there is an important distinction between human rights violations and corruption. Genocide, for example, involves a profound violation of human rights; but it is not corruption. However, there is often a close and mutually reinforcing nexus between corruption and human rights violations, as seen for example in the endemic corruption and large-scale human rights abuses under authoritarian regimes such as those of Idi Amin in Uganda, and Suharto in Indonesia. Or take case study 13.1. This was a case of corruption of institutional processes, including fraud. However, it was also a violation of the human right to life of those haemophiliacs who died as a consequence of being infected by the tainted blood.

Moral judgments, including those in relation to corruption, are not simply expressions of emotion or cases of moralising. Moral judgments can be and often are based on objective evidence, and sometimes made with certainty or near certainty. Consider the claim that the Rwandan genocide was morally wrong. The truth-supporting reasons for this claim include empirical evidence (such as the dead, mutilated bodies of tens of thousands of men, women and children), and moral claims (such as that it is morally wrong to kill innocent people). No rational, morally sentient, person doubts the truth of such moral judgments.

Consider the claims that:

- corrupt judges who enable guilty Mafia bosses to go free ought to be punished; or

- police fabricating evidence against suspects is corruption, and ought not be tolerated; or

- the guilty, but not the innocent, ought to suffer punishment.

Claims such as these are presupposed by entire legal systems.

Definition of corruption

There are a number of related and influential narrow definitions of corruption (Miller 2005, Miller et al 2005). For example, corruption has been characterised as the abuse of power by a public official for private gain. But when police fabricate evidence out of a misplaced sense of justice this is corruption of a public office, but not for private gain. And when a punter bribes a boxer to 'throw' a fight this is corruption for private gain, but it does not necessarily involve any public office holder; the roles of boxer and punter are not necessarily public offices. Or consider a 'gold-digger' who marries a lonely, wealthy man for his money, and thereby deceives him and subverts the purposes of marriage as a social institution.

If an action is corrupt then it corrupts something or someone; so corruption is not only a moral concept, it is a *causal* concept. An action is corrupt only if it has a *corrupting effect* on a person's moral character, or a corrupting effect on an institution.

If an action has a corrupting effect on a person's character, it will typically be corrosive of one or more of a person's virtues, for example, impartiality in a judge or objectivity in a journalist. If an action has a corrupting effect on an institution, then it has a corrupting effect on institutional processes and purposes, and/or on persons in institutional roles. (See for example, case study 13.4.)

On this moral/causal account of corruption an infringement of a specific law or institutional rule does not in and of itself constitute an act of corruption. In order to do so, any such infringement needs to have an institutional *effect*, such as defeating the institutional purpose of the rule, subverting the institutional process governed by the rule, or contributing to the despoiling of the moral character of the role occupant.

If an action is corrupt then the person who performed it either did so intentionally, or he or she performed it knowing the institutional harm it would cause. Or, at the very least, the person could and should have foreseen the harm it would cause. So we should distinguish acts of corruption from acts of institutional *corrosion*. An act might undermine an institutional process or purpose without the person who performed it intending this effect, foreseeing this effect, or indeed even being in a position such that they should have foreseen this effect. Such a deed may well be an act of corrosion, but it would not be an act of corruption. Putting poorly trained judges on the bench may corrode the quality of judiciary, but would not simply in virtue of that be corrupt.

Moreover, those who become corrupted did not necessarily intend their actions to have the effect of corrupting them, nor did they necessarily foresee that they would be corrupted by their actions, and perhaps they could not reasonably have been expected to foresee that they would become corrupted. For example, a child whose parents are fraudsters might become corrupted.

We need to distinguish the following:

1) persons who corrupt (corruptors);
2) persons who are corrupted;
3) acts of corrosion;
4) acts that do not corrupt, but are the expression of a corrupt character, for example, a failed attempt to bribe.

The notion of such a corrupt action presupposes a prior notion of an uncorrupted, and morally legitimate, institution, or institutional process, role or purpose. The act of corruption contributes to bringing about a corrupt condition of some institution.

Consider the uncorrupted judicial process. It consists of the presentation of objective evidence that has been gathered lawfully, of testimony in court being presented truthfully, of the rights of the accused being respected, and so on. To present fabricated evidence, to lie on oath, and so on, are all corrupt actions. An honest accountant who begins to 'doctor the books' under the twin pressures of a corrupt senior management and a desire to maintain an extravagant lifestyle undermines his disposition to act honestly. Consider case studies 13.5 and 13.6. Was Leuci corrupted by the pressures on him? Will Bill be compromised by being promoted by a corrupt boss?

The undermining of institutional processes, roles and purposes, would typically require a pattern of actions, and not merely a single one-off action. There are, however, some single, one-off acts of corruption. One bribe is offered and accepted, and the tendering process is thereby undermined; this is the first and only time that the person offering the bribe and the person receiving the bribe are involved in bribery.

The causal definition is a highly generic definition of corruption. The set of corrupt actions is very wide. They comprise the range of moral and/or legal offences that contribute under certain conditions to despoiling the moral character of persons and/or to undermining morally legitimate institutions. Such offences include:

- bribery, fraud, or nepotism;
- breaches of confidentiality that compromise investigations;
- the making of false statements that undermine court proceedings or selection committee processes or the earned reputations of public figures; and
- selective enforcement of laws or rules by those in authority.

Noble cause corruption

Many motives for corrupt actions exist, including desires for wealth, status, and power. But some actions that are done out of a desire to achieve good are corrupt actions. These are acts of so-called noble cause corruption (Miller 2005, Miller et al 2005), such as fabricating evidence against a known paedophile (as in case study 13.7).

In most cases of noble cause corruption – contra what the person who performs the action thinks – the 'corrupt' action morally ought not be performed. The person who performs the action wrongly believes that he or she is doing the right thing. Nevertheless, *some* acts of noble cause corruption may be morally justified. Suppose I bribe an immigration official to ensure that my friend, who is ineligible to enter Australia, can do so, and thereby have access to life-saving hospital treatment. Surely, I owe it to my friend to save her life, if I can, albeit at the relatively minor moral cost of a one-off act of bribery.

Consider a police officer in India whose meagre wages are insufficient to enable him to feed, clothe and educate his family, and who is prohibited by law from having a second job. So he supplements his income by accepting bribes from certain households in a wealthy area in return for providing additional surveillance and thus greater protection from theft. This has the consequence that other wealthy households tend to suffer a somewhat higher level of theft than otherwise would be the case. This is clearly a case of corruption, indeed noble cause corruption. Arguably, however, given the police officer's moral obligations to his family and the relatively minor degree of harm caused to the wealthy households, his bribe-taking is, all things considered, morally justifiable, or at least morally excusable.

The Watergate break-in was an act of corruption, and – assuming Richard Nixon, Gordon Liddy et al, were motivated by a desire to further the national interest – perhaps an act of noble cause corruption. However, this instance of corruption, indeed of noble cause corruption, was clearly not morally justified. (Consider in this connection case study 13.7. Was it morally justified?)

Machiavelli, Max Weber, Michael Walzer and others have claimed that there is something special about the role of some professions (for example, police, soldiers and political leaders), such that engaging in noble cause corruption is somehow a defining feature of these roles. These theorists are making a stronger claim than that in politics, policing or in the military, as elsewhere, there may well be morally justified acts of noble cause corruption. It is claimed that people in these roles have to accept that they will have 'dirty hands'. The idea is that political leaders, and perhaps the members of some other occupations such as soldiers and police officers, necessarily perform actions that infringe central or important principles of common morality, and that this is because of some inherent feature of these occupations. Such 'dirty' actions include lying, betrayal, and especially violence.

Some putatively 'dirty' actions are indeed definitive of political roles, as they are of police and military roles. For example, a defining feature of police work is its use of harmful and normally immoral methods, such as deceit and violence, in the service of the protection of (among other things) human rights. Such use of deceit and violence is morally justified in terms of the publicly sanctioned, legally enshrined, ethical principles underlying police and military use of harmful and normally immoral methods, including the use of deadly force (Miller, Blackler and Alexandra 2006).

According to Walzer (1973), politicians get their hands dirty by necessity, and he offers two examples. In his first example, a politician in order to get re-elected must make a crooked deal and award contracts to a ward boss. In his second example, a political leader must order the torture of a terrorist leader if he is to discover the whereabouts of bombs planted by the leader and set to go off killing innocent people.

The first example presupposes a corrupt political environment of a kind that in a liberal democracy ought to be opposed and extinguished rather than complied with. Moreover, it is far from clear why the politician's re-election is an overriding moral imperative. The second example is hardly an illustration of what politicians in liberal democracies routinely face. Indeed, even in the context of the so-called war on terror, such cases only arise very occasionally, if at all.

There might be *some* political contexts in which central or important moral principles do need to be infringed on a *routine* basis, albeit for a limited period of time. Consider the use of assassination teams by the Colombian government in its attempts to wrest back control of the country during the period of the drug lord Pablo Escobar. The situation was one of emergency, albeit institutional emergency. So we are not entitled to generalise to other non-emergency political contexts.

Many of the above-described dirty methods, for example, execution and use of criminals to combat criminals – or at least the extent of their usage – were in fact counter-productive. For example, use of other criminal groups against Escobar tended to empower those groups.

Such methods although 'dirty' are not as dirty as can be. Methods such as execution of drug lords are directed at morally culpable persons, as opposed to innocent persons. The dirty end of the spectrum of dirty methods that might be used in politics comprises those methods that involve the intentional harming of innocent persons.

Even if such dirty methods are morally justified their proponents state that their use is necessary. Their aim, they argue, is to re-establish political and other institutions in which the use of such dirty methods would presumably not be permitted. Such scenarios do not demonstrate that the use of dirty methods is a necessary feature of political leadership.

Readings

Daley, Robert (2005) *Prince of the City*, Moyer Bell, Kingston, pp 124–25.

Larmour, Peter and Wolanin, Nick (eds) (2000) *Corruption and Anti-corruption*, Asia-Pacific Press, Canberra.

Machiavelli, Niccolò (1513, 1981) *The Prince*, Penguin, Harmondsworth.

McCarthy, Bernard J (1991) 'Keeping an eye on the keeper: Prison corruption and its control' in Braswell, Michael, McCarthy, Belinda R and McCarthy, Bernard J (eds) *Justice, Crime and Ethics*, Anderson, Cincinnati, p 248.

Miller, Seumas (2005) 'Corruption', *Stanford Encyclopedia of Philosophy*, Summer.

Miller, Seumas, Blackler, John and Alexandra, Andrew (2006) *Police Ethics*, 2nd ed, Allen & Unwin, Sydney.

Miller, Seumas, Roberts, Peter and Spence, Edward (2005) *Corruption and Anti-corruption*, Prentice Hall, Upper Saddle River, pp 103–04.

Thompson, Dennis (1995) *Ethics in Congress: From Individual to Institutional Corruption*, Brookings Institute, Washington DC.

Walzer, Michael (1973) 'Political action: The problem of dirty hands', *Philosophy and Public Affairs*, vol 2, no 2, Winter.

Weber, Max (1919) 'Politics as a vocation', available at <http://www.ne.jp/asahi/moriyuki/abukuma/weber/lecture/politics_vocation.html> (accessed 2/2/09).

Wueste, Daniel E (ed) (1994) *Ethics and Social Responsibility*, Rowman and Littlefield, Lanham MD, pp 15–16.

Index

family, institution of 215, 217 *see also* family, institution of

filial responsibility, not enshrined in law 227 *see also* filial responsibility

homicides in families 219

immigration official, bribe of 267

IVF legally prohibited for single women in Victoria 196 *see also* ART

liberty rights 190

population, ageing 216

population, policy to increase 192 *see also* public policy

primary school education 190 *see also* education

Prime Minister John Howard 197 *see also* ART

suicide 163

'White Australia' policy 174

autonomy 3, 26–27, 127–30, 134, 135, 153, 164, 168, 171–72, 228, 246–47 *see also* drug addiction; duty of care; filial responsibility; informed consent; paternalism; right to die

and desire to do what is forbidden 85–86

and rationality 136

and right to life 134

and solitary confinement 246–47

application of term 129–30, 131

as both rational and moral 127–28

as condition for other goods 247

constraints on autonomy 129

degrees of autonomy 130

diminished autonomy 247

independence necessary for autonomy 128

non-rational/irrational and non-moral/ immoral agents 128

rational/moral distinction 127–28

beliefs 127 *see also* cultural relativism; moral beliefs

beneficence (helping others) 133 *see also* paternalism

cannibalism 17–18, 21, 79 *see also* cultural relativism

choice 27, 46, 129, 136–37, 176, 246

character and choice 67–68

compassion 83, 87, 165–66, 171 *see also* death; life; moral emotion

confidentiality, professional 101–102, 105, 147–51 *see also* privacy; privacy and confidentiality, case studies

breaches of confidentiality 266

confidentiality and HIV 150–51

confidentiality and professional

effectiveness/morality 151

confidentiality derived from notion of privacy 151–52, 153–54

confidentiality non-absolute 147–48, 150

necessary to preserve trust (trust argument) 149–51

where necessary for harm prevention 149

moral justification for confidentiality 147, 150

trust 147, 150 *see also* duty of care

confidentiality, varieties of 148

client/practitioner confidentiality 147, 148–4, 154

conscience 86

corruption 8, 260–69

as corrosive of virtues 264

corruption of public officials (Prohibition) 248–49

many offence types are corruption 262

moral judgments in relation to corruption 263

corruption, definition of 264–66

as abuse of power 264

as matter of morality not law 262–63

causal definition of corruption 264, 266

corrupt actions and immoral actions 263

corrupt actions not necessarily unlawful actions 262

corruptors/corrupted and corrosion/ corrupt character distinctions 265

human rights violations/corruption distinction 263

corruption, institutional 262, 264

specific law/rule infringement not corruption 264

institutional corruption/corrosion 265

corrupt action presupposes uncorrupted institution 265–66

pattern of corrupt actions not one-off action 266

corruption, noble cause 266–69

as defining feature of some professions 267–68

deadly force, use of 268

'dirty hands' 267–69

most noble cause corruption not justified 266–67

some noble cause corruption morally justified 267

corruption, noble cause, examples 266–69

assassination teams, Colombia (Pablo Escobar) 268–69

police officer in India accepting bribes 267

political leader orders torture of terrorist 268